Child Care:
Some Nursing Perspectives

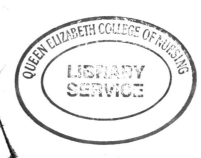

Child Care: Some Nursing Perspectives

Edited by Alan Glasper

A collection of articles first published in Professional Nurse and here revised and updated, with additional articles specially commissioned for inclusion

Wolfe Publishing Ltd

Published by
Wolfe Publishing Ltd
Brook House
2–16 Torrington Place
London WC1E 7LT

Printed by BPCC Hazell Books, Aylesbury, England.

© 1991 Wolfe Publishing

ISBN 1 8700 6523 9

For full details of all Wolfe Nursing titles please write to Wolfe
Publishing Ltd, Brook House, 2–16 Torrington Place, London
WC1E 7LT, England.

The Professional Developments Series

These eight books provide you with a wealth of insight into all aspects of nursing practice. The series is essential reading for qualified, practising nurses who need to keep up-to-date with new developments, evaluate their clinical practice, and develop and extend their clinical management and teaching skills. Through reading these books, students of nursing will gain an insight into what the essence of nursing is and the wide range of skills which are daily employed in improving patient care. Up-to-date, referenced and appropriately illustrated, The Professional Developments Series brings together the work of well over two hundred nurses.

Other titles in The Professional Developments Series:

Dunne   **How Many Nurses Do I Need: A Guide**   1 870065 24 7
to Resource Management Issues
This book provides valuable advice and information for all nurses facing the challenge of taking direct responsibility for managing human resources and planning, providing quality assurance and managing financial resources.

Garrett   **Healthy Ageing: Some Nursing Perspectives**   1 870065 22 0
This book puts healthy ageing into the context of a growing, healthy elderly population and looks at care aspects of daily living, health problems in old age, and working with older people.

Horne   **Effective Communication**   1 870065 14 X
This book examines a wide range of communication topics, including counselling, confidentiality, group and team work, compliance and communicating with children.

Horne   **Patient Education Plus**   1 870065 11 5
This book helps to develop nurses' teaching roles, and covers an extensive range of clinical topics. Each chapter contains a useful handout which can be freely photocopied or adapted for use with clients.

Horne   **Practice Check!**   1 870065 10 7
Each Practice Check presents a brief description of situations which may arise in practice together with open-ended questions and discussion to enable problems to be explored and effective solutions to be found.

Horne   **Staff Nurse's Survival Guide**   1 870065 13 1
Relevant to recently qualified and experienced nurses working in all healthcare settings, this brings together chapters on a wide range of clinical and non-clinical issues in patient care.

Horne   **Ward Sister's Survival Guide**   1 870065 12 3
This book is essential reading and a valuable reference for all nurses with direct clinical management responsibility.

Contents

Adolescence: Health Concerns

Hospital and Illness: A Child's Perspective

Introduction

Rachael Smith, RGN, RSCN, Dip N (Lond), RNT, PGCEA
Senior Tutor, Child Health, Southampton University College of Nursing

Nurses in the 1990s work in a climate of tremendous change. Unfortunately, not a single change, but several major ones arriving from different origins, interwoven and each having bearing upon the other. As Wilson (1989) remarked "Change is a permanent feature of most organisations and currently a major issue in nursing."

The most remarkable change, with far reaching effects, is the revolution in the management of the NHS contained within the 1990 NHS and Community Care Act. The act is the evidence of the government's resolve to tackle the "underlying problems in the management and funding of the NHS . . . (and) to increase the efficiency with which resources are used." (Ham, 1990).

Major reforms are in process in relation to preregistration nurse education which arose from the UKCC (1986) Project 2000 paper, reflecting the professions desire to address many important issues and to take nursing into the 20th century. Project 2000 courses call for new approaches, changed attitudes and are very demanding on all concerned in providing nurse education. The potential for a degree of unease and uncertainty for clinical colleagues and educational staff as these challenges are met are obvious.

Following close on the heels of preregistration changes are the proposed changes in the UKCC Post-Registration Education and Practice Project (PREPP) document, with many of the profession divided on the strengths of the proposals.

The nurse of today caring for children does not stand alone in marrying the philosophies of care delivery to a distinct client group. The role of these nurses is to meet the unique needs of, and to provide quality care for, the child and family within a hospital and community setting. The role is an evolutionary one which, by its very nature of adaptation and elements of challenge, may be uncomfortable. Amongst the many qualities required of today's practitioner and in particular the successful manager are ". . . charisma, managerial skills, ability to inspire others with a vision of a better future and to handle the practicality of attaining it. Simply to manage and to maintain the *status quo* is no longer enough." (Salvage, 1989).

Changes in practice

Caring for the child and family has dramatically changed over the last three decades. The thrust for these changes has come from many quarters including the Platt Report (1959), and the Court Report (1976). Both reports were long, in-depth studies of the provisions for children in hospital and although in essence many of the recommendations of the reports were very similar, the Court Report has had greater impact on practice being changed. The fifteen year time gap may well have been influential in this respect.

The National Association of the Welfare of Children in Hospital (NAWCH) has, and continues to be, a moving force in highlighting, researching and recommending improved practice. Other invaluable research is being undertaken by a joint committee Caring for Children in the Health Services and several important reports have been published by this committee. The latest, *Just For The Day* (Thornes, 1991) is an excellent tool for evaluating provisions for day care and initiating development in such an important aspect of care provision within the new NHS structure.

The role of parents   An example of change in the philosophy of child care, which has moved through a gradual transitional period, is in relation to the role of parents in care. I personally have vivid memories of being in hospital as a child where a very restricted, parents-only, visiting policy was adhered to. Later as a paediatric student nurse in the late 1960s, parents were tolerated but not actively encouraged to participate in care.

With gradual relaxation of visiting regulations and a greater part played by parents in the care of the sick child there has been a corresponding shift from a more institutional style of care to a family centred philosophy. Family centred care defines the focus of paediatric care, that being, the whole family. It provides the opportunity for the family to care for the hospitalised child under nursing supervision.

A next step in the care of some children in hospital is a concept which emerged in the late 1960s and early 1970s in North America and Canada, 'Care by Parent Units'. The care by parent philosophy defines a three way partnership where doctors, parents and nurses unite towards a common, shared goal, that being the best care for the child and family. To transform this vision into a working reality requires insight, innovation and a genuine commitment to accept the implicit changes in role function. Detailed planning and implementation is vital as well as evaluation of this approach to care delivery.

Parents continue to provide care after the child is discharged from hospital highlighting another very important area of change, that being the role of the community nurse. With the introduction and increase of day care provision, decreased length of hospital stay with earlier discharge, and the provision of care to children who would previously have been confined to hospital, the demands of a community nursing service to meet the needs of the child and family has evolved. Whilst some Health Authorities recognise the need for a paediatric nursing community service, others lag sadly behind.

Yet further legislation which came into effect in October 1991, The Children Act, has profound bearing on provision of care and as such must be taken on board by paediatric nurses. One of the principle intentions of the act is to address the balance between the duty to protect children and the need to give parents more opportunity to be involved in decisions. There are implied changes in practice to virtually all professional groups coming into contact with children.

Care educator and supporter Within the many spheres of child nursing the effects of change upon role and responsibility is evident. A reflection of this is embodied by the following quote. "Paediatric nurses are required to shed their traditional role as primary care giver and adapt a new role of care educator and supporter to parents as they continue their role as primary care givers" (Gibson 1989).

Caring for clients in the 1990s demands a professional nurse who is a competent, accountable practitioner who is able to deliver skilled care to the child and family at all ages, developmental stages and levels of dependency in a variety of settings.

Problem-solver and innovator Amongst the many skills required are the ability to problem solve and be creative and innovative in areas of potential improvement for care. Practice must be based on a sound awareness and utilization of research and the professional carer must be able to contribute to the developing body of knowledge through research. The opportunities for promoting optimum health and the prevention of ill-health are challenges to be met and necessitate a high degree of teaching skills. The paediatric nurse of the 1990s must be able to act as an equal and complimentary member of the multidisciplinary team in many settings.

References
Court, S.D.M. (1976) *Fit for the Future*. Report of the Committee on Child Health Services. Volume I and II. HMSO, London.
Gibson, F. (1989) Parental involvement in bone marrow transplant. *Paediatric Nursing*, **1**, (1).
Ham, C. (1990) *The New National Health Service Organisation and Management*. Radcliffe Medical Press, Oxford.
Platt, H. (1959) *The Welfare of Children in Hospital*. Report of the Committee on Child Health Services. HMSO London.
Salvage, J. (1989) Take me to your Leader. *Nursing Times*, June 21.
The Children Act (1989) HMSO, London.
Thornes, R. (1991) *Just For The Day*. NAWCH, London.
Tucker, A. (1990) Preparing for Practice. *Paediatric Nursing*. Vol II No. 1.
UKCC (1986) *Project 2000: A New Preparation For Practice*. UKCC, London.
UKCC (1991) *Post-Registration Education and Practice Project*. UKCC, London.
Wilson, J. (1989) The shifting sands of management. *Senior Nurse*, **9**, (7).

Aspects of Neonatal Care

1

Dilemmas in neonatal units

Alison J. Stewart, RGN, RM, RHV, MSc
Research Midwife, Bristol Maternity Hospital

The cost in time and effort needed to care for babies in a neonatal unit (NNU) can obscure some of the dilemmas common to this area of work. Nurses may find themselves in a situation where personal values conflict with professional actions. Staff may suffer from unresolved conflict and stress, surviving at great personal cost and at the risk of suffering burnout.

Ethical dilemmas

The question at the heart of the debate on the intensive care of neonates is who to treat and who not to treat? There are various facets to this problem.

- Assuming infinite resources, should the existence of technology mean it should automatically be offered to all babies? The development of sophisticated equipment and surgical techniques has meant babies who would previously have died are now surviving. However, the conditions of survival raise many questions. If we accept that some babies will require long-term treatment and follow-up, that others will be handicapped, marriages may be broken and parents depressed – is the cost too great? The arguments for the use of selective or universal treatment are as follows:
- It has been suggested that a baby is not a person – defined as having the ability to perceive one's own future and an awareness of self. Singer (1979) wrote, "killing a defective infant is not morally equivalent to killing a person". Is this acceptable? Are babies people with rights?
- Alternatively, there is the issue of quality of life as a result of treatment. How do we decide on a derived measure of life acceptable to child and family? Long-term follow-up studies provide data on which to base some decisions. For babies of birth weight less than 1,000g, morbidity rates (eg, cerebral palsy) have been found in the range of 25–50 per cent (Ovgill *et al*, 1982; Hernandez *et al*, 1986; Sandhu *et al*, 1986). What about social /emotional sequelae?
- From a religious basis, the sanctity of life may require doing the utmost to preserve and save life. Can this be extended too far? What is life? Does it include cerebral aspects or is it based purely on physiological processes?

- From a utilitarian point of view, the cost to society to treat these children is out of all proportion to the future contribution they may make. This may appear harsh, but then it is society that pays the cost of care for a lifetime.
- From a scientific point of view, the use of aggressive treatment has been justified as necessary to further advance knowledge and expertise to save more children in the future. Is there any limit to this or are we seeking to ultimately develop technology to act as an artificial placenta? This has Orwellian overtones of 1984, with the whole process of childbearing becoming mechanised.

Discriminatory use of treatment

A major aspect of the medical/nursing role has always been the challenge to combat death – the desire to be omnipotent and to alter the outcome. This tends to apply principally to the indiscriminatory use of treatment. How does the fact that the patient is a baby affect the argument? It may introduce emotive overtones that it is 'cruel' and 'unfair' either to let the baby suffer or not to treat. Increasingly, paediatricians and nurses appear to be questioning the consequences of their care. In a World in Action programme, a Manchester doctor indicated he was prepared to withdraw treatment rather than artificially prolong a life which would have little subsequent quality or potential.

The decision not to resuscitate or treat is fraught with ethical and legal pit-holes, since technically it may be interpreted as either murder, manslaughter or compassionate good sense. This explains why staff approach this area with such caution, particularly in view of the defensive medicine practised in the US.

Who decides?　If we allow that some sort of decision should be made about which babies to treat – who makes that decision? It could be at Government level creating legal criteria, at hospital level with a particular unit policy, or at the individual level of clinicians and parents. Any discriminatory decisions need both medical and nursing agreement, otherwise nurses can feel increasingly stressed and embittered at their exclusion from the decision-making process while still being expected to provide 24-hour care beside the cot (Savage, 1988).

What of the parents' role in this decision? It is, after all, their baby. Savage (1988) found the majority of nurses (92.6 per cent) felt parents should participate in any do not resuscitate (DNR) decision. However, a World in Action programme (1988) has illustrated that some parents feel it impossible or inappropriate to do so (either because they lack sufficient understanding of the medical situation or they are too involved). Others feel it is their right to determine the outcome for their child. If a baby dies, then its parents need careful counselling to help them come to terms with their baby's death and any potential feelings of guilt.

How to decide?   If decisions are made about whether or not to continue treatment, what are the criteria? Whitelaw (1986) wrote about "death as an option". In a four year period at the Hammersmith Hospital, London, 30 per cent of deaths occurred after withdrawal of treatment. The decision was "based on a virtual certainty, not just of handicap but of total incapacity eg, microcephaly". There can be considerable difficulty in determining criteria, since the situation of each baby (gestation, handicap, clinical problems) and family reaction will vary drastically. At Hammersmith, the decision had to be unanimous among staff, with parental agreement.

Paradoxical infanticide?   The fact that treatment withdrawn on a 26-week baby in NNU might constitute murder, whereas therapeutic termination of pregnancy (TOP) of a similar gestation fetus is legal, makes a farce of the situation. The existing limit of 28 weeks for TOP dates from when the expected viability of a fetus was upwards of this gestation. Various attempts to reduce the legal limit have failed eg, Alton 1987/88. Currently, an unspoken agreement exists among gynaecologists not to perform late abortions (26-28 weeks), since, as obstetricians, they are delivering babies of the same age in maternity units. As nurses providing 24-hour care in both situations, how do we reconcile this anomalous state of affairs, and what are the everyday effects on our work and behaviour?

Money and resources

The dilemma of who to treat is further exacerbated by the inadequate resources available to meet the demands of a rising neonatal population. A recent report by the Royal College of Physicians (1988) estimated that 2,000 preterm babies are dying each year because of a shortage of cots, equipment and staff. What role do *in vitro* fertilisation programmes and infertility treatment have in overstretching a service which is already at bursting point? A set of preterm triplets or quads may swamp a NNU, taking over most of the ventilators and equipment and blocking cots for weeks or months. Should more rigid controls/quotas exist in view of limited resources?

Treatment tends to be allocated on an *ad hoc*, first-come-first-served basis until there is full cot occupancy. It is impossible to refuse the last empty cot to a 26-week baby on the basis that a 30-week baby might deliver which would be a better bet in terms of cost-benefit outcome. Newns *et al* (1984) estimated that the average cost for survivors was £5,500 with birthweight 1-1.5kg and £10,000 birthweight <1kg.

The existence of new life-saving technology can create demands for it to be universally available. However, NHS resources have always been finite and, to some degree, this has enforced a situation of healthcare rationing. Without definitive guidelines, resources become increasingly overstretched, resulting in universal suboptimal care. The consequent morbidity can then have long-term costs for both family and state (Murton et al, 1987).

Monetary aspects aside, nursing staff shortages and long hours on call for doctors have detrimental effects on existing staff who end up coping against all odds; this can lead to loss of job satisfaction, increasing stress and even burnout. In addition, the difficulty in recruiting a full complement of staff may mean the unit is always below full-cot occupancy, having to refuse care and refer babies elsewhere. How does this look to managers with figures on paper revealing failure to fully utilise resources? The danger is that emergency situations may cause yet another baby to be squeezed in, placing staff in the invidious position of feeling compelled to push themselves further to care for an extra patient. How does this type of situation affect morale?

Nurse as advocate

Nurses may act as a buffer between doctor and parents, and if both have opposing views on the care of the baby they may feel torn in two. For example, parents may view treatment as 'cruel' and loudly express their feelings or even refuse to countenance necessary actions, such as Jehovah's Witnesses refusing blood transfusions for a baby incapacitated by anaemia. In these sort of situations, it is vital that open communication is established: support groups to air views and the presence of someone trained in counselling techniques are invaluable.

Nurses can also be caught between doctors and the baby, acting as the baby's advocate – for example, stopping medical staff from losing a sense of perspective and fighting on to try and site an IV cannula when the baby is exhausted. Alternatively, it may involve campaigning for pain relief, which is rarely administered even following major surgery or prior to procedures such as siting an umbilical catheter or an IV cannula. There appears to be an implicit assumption that babies do not feel pain because they can only feebly protest and grimace, unlike a vocal adult. It may cause nurses considerable distress to realise the majority of their care constitutes a series of assaults, as endotracheal tubes are sucked out and electrodes resited. The majority of babies have behavioural or physiological changes (eg, cry, move or tachycardia) in response to these actions, which can be perceived as their way of expressing pain.

Coping with failure

The aim of medical/nursing care is to win against the odds – save lives and restore health; it is by these criteria that we measure general and personal performance. To have a patient die or just to offer tender loving care can appear as an admission of failure. It is hard to sit back, be peaceful and not to use available aggressive treatment; we are not taught to accept the sense of helplessness this engenders. The situation is exacerbated when caring for a small baby since there are inevitable emotional overtones – he or she is only just born and has had no chance to see life. The strain of coping with our own reactions, and being involved in the family situation can be enormous and lead to a sense of failure.

The media headlines and public expectations of the 'miracles' of NNUs may create a constant demand which we may feel we have to live up to. The public is not always aware of the long, slow haul from birth to discharge with the accompanying strain and tension on family and staff. Such pressures make it harder for staff in NNUs to accept the loss of babies and the failure of not achieving a 100 per cent success rate.

The age-old complaint of having insufficient time to achieve standards set, such as talking to parents or keeping up with an endless round of observations and care, is exacerbated by staff shortages. The dilemma of what to compromise on and what cannot be realistically achieved in the time available can cause distress and loss of job satisfaction. When this occurs, it needs to be brought to the attention of managers who may either revise expectations or employ more staff or reduce cot-occupancy. There is no point in sitting tight and muttering, in the end it is the families and staff who suffer.

The work of neonatal nurses tends to be concentrated on painfully emotional issues: death and dying; sickness and health; disability and handicap. As nurses we may find it difficult to resolve our feelings and seek to subvert or deny them rather than recognise, confront and work them through. In our training and in life we are not taught to grieve and accept loss and change.

Support groups

Units are increasingly using support group sessions for staff with or without parents, often with a trained counsellor present. This offers the opportunity to share feelings and frustrations and can give a valuable insight into how others cope and respond. However, there is always the problem of how far to expose oneself to the public gaze of colleagues, particularly if our comments and ideas are not acceptable or the unit norm. How far do we trust each other and how honest can we be? This is one of the reasons why support groups are unpopular and not perceived as constructive. Only when we are comfortable with ourselves can we hope to face some of the emotions and reactions that devastated parents may exhibit. These may include aggression, anger and physical violence directed at all carers. It requires skill and self-confidence to defuse and restructure these type of situations to a constructive ending.

To survive and enjoy an intensive care situation as nurses, we need to develop our ideas and conclusions about the implicit dilemmas confronting us. By doing this, we will be contributing to our development as a mature profession with informed accountability for our actions and with stable, well-balanced dispositions!

References

Burnard, P. (1988) Coping with other people's emotions. *The Professional Nurse*, **4**, 1, 11–14.

Hernandez, J.A., Offut, J. and Butterfield, L.J. (1986) The cost of care of the less than 1000gm infants. *Clin. Perinatology*, **13**, 461–76.

Murton, L. *et al* (1987) Care of VLBW infants with limited neonatal intensive care resources. *Medical Journal of Australia*, Jan. 19, 46, 78–81.

Newns, B. *et al* (1984) Costs and outcomes in a regional neonatal ICU. *Arch. Dis. Child*, **59**, 11, 1064–7.

Ovgill, A.A. *et al* (1982) Early development of infants of 1000gm or less at birth. *Arch. Dis. Child.*, **57**, 11, 823–7.

Report by the Royal College of Physicians (1988). Care of the Newborn in England and Wales, RCP, London.

Sandhu, B. *et al* (1986) Cost of neonatal intensive care for VLBW infants. *Lancet*, **1**, March 15, 600–3.

Singer, P. (1979) Practical Ethics. Cambridge University Press, Cambridge.

World in Action. HTV, Oct. 3, 1988.

Bibliography

Penticuff, J.H. (1987) Neonatal nursing ethics: towards a consensus. *Neonatal Network*, **5**, 6, 7–16.

Although applying to American NNUs, makes very useful reading on a variety of issues and stresses the importance of nurses becoming involved in ethical decisions.

Richards, M. (1987) The withdrawal of treatment from newborn infants. MIDIRS information pack No. 5, August, Postnatal section.

Discussion of issues in the withdrawing of treatment.

2

Mums and dads need care too: supporting parents of babies in neonatal units

Alison J. Stewart, RGN, RM, RHV, MSc
Research Midwife, Bristol Maternity Hospital

Becoming a parent can be a time of crisis, with severe emotional upset and tension, while pregnancy is a transition period from independence to being responsible for the nurture of a helpless being. LeMasters (1979) found that 83 per cent of parents rated the arrival of their first child as a crisis event. The main problems cited were 'unpreparedness' for the realities of caring for a baby, such as tiredness, coping with feeds and a crying baby, all of which tend to be minimised by the romantic media image of perfect parenthood, with the cooing and chubby baby. For women the period of upset and confusion is heightened by the physical strain of labour and the changes which occur in the puerperium. Caplan (1965) has argued that life crises occur when a state of disequilibrium occurs and that for parents this is normally a short-term state as role readjustment occurs.

The arrival of the anticipated normal, healthy baby can be a positive event and do much to ease the adjustment of roles and ideas, but parents whose baby requires admission to a neonatal unit (NNU) do not have the comfort of cuddling their baby whenever they wish, helping them to perceive themselves as parents. For these parents the predominant feelings may be negative and long-lasting: aggression, anxiety, frustration, shock, fear, confusion, guilt and failure at the need for admission and the separation from their baby (McGovern, 1984; Alderson, 1983). Each parent is an individual and will bring a different set of beliefs, fears and needs with them. One of the main difficulties for parents is finding out what their role is in a NNU. How fulfilled they feel and how developed that role is depends on the staff.

As a visitor?
Twenty years ago, parental entry to NNUs was severely restricted and subject to staff dictates, in an attempt to avoid cross-infection. Parents were cast in the role of visitors, with the connotation of being invited and grudgingly allowed in, rather than having a right to come and go at will. The situation has now radically altered, due to staff awareness and the

efforts of pressure groups such as National Association for the Welfare of Children in Hospital (NAWCH), and most units now have 'open' visiting – 24 hours per day (Thornes, 1985). Encouragement and explanation can familiarise parents and help them to feel less like intruders, as can facilities to make them more comfortable, such as kitchen, toilets and television, and the availability of information leaflets.

Parents as carers

Increasingly we are seeing families as 'healthcare agencies' responsible for the provision and maintenance of the health of its members. As Price (1987) notes, this can involve various functions: protecting and nurturing; lay care partners assisting professionals; pressure groups on behalf of the patient.

Normally, after the child is born, parents assume the responsibility for meeting his or her needs, such as feeding, changing and cuddling. Babies admitted to NNUs are separated from their parents, whose role as parents and providers is demeaned or totally negated, making them feel useless. They may see their child as belonging to medical/nursing staff and be too awed, frightened or overwhelmed by the surroundings to suggest that they become involved in providing care. Staff in NNUs need to take the initiative to suggest various ways in which parents can care for their baby (Table 1) to enhance their self-esteem as parents, which may be severely damaged by the birth of a baby who is not 'perfect'. Caring

---

- Cuddling the baby – providing comfort and contact.
- Feeding the baby – tube/breast/bottle.
- Choosing or providing milk, eg humilacting breast milk or deciding on a particular brand.
- Nappy changing/cord care.
- Cleaning the baby's mouth with moist cotton wool buds if not on oral feeds.
- Removing phototherapy goggles during nappy care.
- Stroking/massaging the baby's head.
- Putting toys, photos or pictures in the incubator/cot.
- Bringing the baby's own clothes and dressing him/her.
- Assisting nursing staff, handing items as needed, steadying tubes/probes when changing the baby's position or sheets.
- Maintaining a weight/progress chart and photographic record of changes.

Table 1. Suggestions for parental involvement in care.

activities also offer opportunities to meet and bond with the baby – separation has been cited as a cause of failure to bond, and early contact can have a long-term beneficial effect (Klaus and Kennell, 1976).

Physical care

The extent to which parents will become involved in the physical care of a baby will depend on parental inclination, unit policy and staff encouragement. For example, some units are happy for parents to perform tube-feeds once they have been safely supervised. However, even within a unit there may be variations between staff in how much they encourage parents to do. Thornes (1985) pointed out that "an inconsistent approach from staff does not encourage confidence. Cases have been reported of mothers who carried out a procedure successfully one day but were prevented from doing the same tasks by a different staff member the following day." A specified unit policy and documented approach of what aspects of care parents can be involved in can reduce this confusion. Care should also be taken to ensure that parents arrive when care is needed; coinciding with the time for observations, feeds and nappy changes: this may be a particular problem once the mother is discharged home, and will require liaison to avoid her making wasted journeys when feed times change.

Feeding the baby, whether by tube, bottle or breast, is often seen as the ultimate expression of care and love. Whatever the method, parents need to be taught how best to do it and given handy hints about baby behaviour, such as dealing with winding and hiccups. Mothers expressing milk for babies who are not currently enterally feeding need considerable support and praise, since it takes considerable effort and determination to continue.

It is equally important for staff on the unit to teach parents how to change nappies and wash their baby's face, since these skills are not instinctive. Any parent, regardless of how many previous children they may have had, tends to welcome a few reminders – and anyone is daunted at the idea of trying to juggle sticky tapes of a nappy inside an incubator. If parents are to feel confident carers they need sufficient support to achieve an appropriate level of competence.

Emotional care

It is vital that parents realise they provide comfort and security for their baby. They need to be taught how to cuddle a baby attached to probes, ECG monitors and drip, and can actively contribute to the baby's emotional development by providing sensory input and stimulation. For example, photos of parents/siblings can be stuck to the incubator or cot at the level of the baby's head so that as he or she turns from side to side the photos are there. Tapes of soft music or parents' voices reading a story might be played in the incubator or nearby, while pieces of sheepskin for the baby to lie on can provide tactile stimulation and warmth, and small toys and mobiles can personalise the area surrounding the baby, making it feel more like home. At the end of the day parents need to feel they are providing the loving touch.

If they are not allowed or encouraged to develop their caring role, the danger exists that parents may have difficulty in assuming or resuming it when the baby gets better and is ready to go home. Some parents find it difficult to believe their baby is judged 'well' and that they are now competent to look after him or her, which may cause ambivalent feelings about taking the baby home (Salitros, 1986). Involving parents in care throughout their baby's stay in hospital can alleviate some of the panic experienced on discharge (Hawthorne, 1984).

Planning for discharge and equipping parents with information and skills to cope at home should be an integral part of neonatal care. However, discharge preparation can be woefully inadequate, and frequently parents are not asked what they wish to know. Marshall (1987) discovered that:

- Skills such as bathing were taught by junior, inexperienced staff with little room for parents to practise themselves.
- Social and psychological preparation appeared to be the most neglected area, such as what to expect in terms of future behaviour and problems.
- Discharge was based on the medical model – that the baby was better, and not on a holistic one of when family and baby were ready.

A consistent, well-planned and documented approach appears necessary for successful discharge, and it may be useful to conduct a survey of parents to find out what they want to know. Many units also have various facilities to aid the transition to home (Table 2).

- Mother and baby rooms in NNUs, where parents 'room in' for several nights prior to discharge and give 24 hour care to the baby while medical/nursing advice and treatment is still on hand.
- Transitional Care Units (TCU) where parents can care for babies in a more homelike setting, with staff available when necessary to perform and advise on care.
- Specialist support (eg, Prem Team midwives) in the community who may visit daily or weekly over a period of weeks or months as necessary. They liaise with the unit, meet the parents prior to discharge and appreciate the needs of these particular babies and families when settling down at home.

Table 2. Facilities to help parents adjust to being carers.

Learning about their baby

As intensive care becomes more complex, the battery of clicking, flashing, whirring and bleeping equipment may be a source of horrified fascination and fear. Seeing a member of the family amidst all this technology can cause emotional crisis (Daley, 1984). The two main expressed wishes of families tend to be:

- that they are informed truthfully of the patient's condition;
- to know the best care is being offered (this may involve nurses in explaining the need for and value of equipment).

This places a considerable onus on staff to provide sufficient explanation and information – and to repeat it, as most parents in a shocked state cannot readily assimilate it initially. In addition to learning what is happening to their baby, parents also need time to come to 'know' their baby. They need to see the child as an individual and to be able to interpret/perceive his or her reactions and needs.

Parents as guardians or advocates

An important aspect of being a parent is to protect children from potentially harmful events. Their capacity on the unit is to represent the best interests of their child and to reflect the needs and wishes of the child if he or she could express them. This means parents should be involved in treatment decisions: frequently they are seen as being too over-wrought to be able to participate intelligently in decisions. Taylor (1986) points out that "Being emotionally troubled does not make parents unintelligent, nor prevent them from using the intelligence they have". The danger is that staff may develop strategies to give information in short bursts and then become engrossed in care of, and procedures with, the baby, thus terminating spontaneous conversation and discussion. This is frequently a consequence of work pressures and may be one of the disadvantages of busy regional units taking all the 'difficult' cases as opposed to the steadier work pace of provincial units.

Parents as part of a family

In an intensive care situation it is easy to focus attention on the critically ill patient and fail to see the family holistically, with an established network of relationships. The involvement of siblings in NNU can reduce the conflicting demands on parents and minimise the sense of alienation or resentment siblings may feel towards the baby as the focus of attention. Involvement can include nappy changes, cuddling the baby and keeping a weight chart.

The clinical, overcrowded environment of NNU is not conducive to lengthy visits from children at any age – the provision of toys, a play area and even a playworker can help make visiting a success.

If they are to effectively care for their baby, all parents need help, which often comes from family, friends and professionals. Numerous reasons may cause parents to need and/or seek counselling, support and just a chance to chat. McHaffie (1987) found in a group of mothers on NNU with a low birthweight baby that all apparently needed "someone who can be quiet and still, who will listen attentively without interfering, who will be comfortable simply to be with rather than preoccupied by doing things". She argues that this is part of the nurse's or midwife's role. However, with current staffing levels there is little time to stop and listen for hours, nor may nurses feel competent to deal with some of the emotions encountered. Sources of help are listed in Table 3.

- Family/social worker – attached to the unit with counselling skills – acts as liaison between parents and staff: his or her job is to have time for the parents.
- Linkworkers/interpreters can be invaluable when communicating with other cultures – to ensure adequate explanation and ascertain any particular religious/cultural requests.
- Chaplains/religious workers may be contacted by nurses and parents to come and visit on the unit and offer comfort – possibly suggest a christening for a very sick baby.
- Psychotherapist referral if one is attached to the unit. Vas Dias (1987) cites the use of techniques to help families come to terms with their baby or his or her death.
- Parent/staff support groups – at an informal level, introductions by staff of mothers to each other, and at a more formal level with organised meetings.
- Contact addresses of people who are willing to 'adopt' parents who may have transferred many miles from home to the facilities available in a regional unit.

Table 3. Sources of help for parents.

One method of particular value to help parents share and express their feelings has been the use of parent or parent-staff support groups. These can be useful sources of comfort and feedback. Otherwise "parents may feel it is inappropriate to criticise one aspect of the care while being so grateful for the clinical care their baby is receiving" (Thornes, 1985).

Parents as members of the unit?

As staff, we need to adopt a positive partnership with parents and make sure we recognise the contribution that they alone can make to their child's wellbeing. Everyone's aim is for the babies on NNUs to recover and to be discharged into the care of confident and competent parents – we are just the facilitators in this process.

References

Alderson, P. (1983) *Special Care for Babies in Hospital*. NAWCH, London.
Caplan, G. (1964) *Principles of Preventive Psychiatry*. Tavistock Publications, London.
Daley, M. (1984) Families in critical care. *Heart and Lung*, **13**, 3, 231–37.
Hawthorne, J. (1984) Support for parents of babies in special care baby units. *Midwives Chronicle*, **97**, 1157, 170–74.
Klaus, M.H. and Kennell, J.H. (1976) *Maternal Infant Bonding*. C.V. Mosby, St. Louis.
LeMasters, E.E. (1979) *Parenthood as a Crisis*. Family Service Association of America, New York.
Marshall, J. (1987) A review of the discharge preparation and initial community support given to families of neonates after surgical intensive care. *Intensive Care Nursing*, **2**, 101–06.

McGovern, M. (1984) Separation of the baby from the parents. *Nursing Times*, **80**, 4, 28-30.
McHaffie, H. (1987) Isolated but not alone. *Nursing Times*, **83**, 28, 73–74.
Price, B. (1987) Happy families. *Nursing Times*, **83**, 47, 45–47.
Salitros, P. (1986) Transitional infant care: a bridge to home for high risk infants. *Neonatal Network*, Feb. 35–41.
Taylor, P. (1986) Promoting parental care of high risk babies. *Aust. Nurses Journal*, **15**, 8, 31–33.
Thornes, R. (1985) Parent participation. *Nursing Mirror*, **160**, 12, 20–22.
Vas Dias, S. (1987) Psychotherapy in SCBU. *Nursing Times*, **83**, 23, 50–52.

Bibliography
Two books which are very readable sources of information aimed at both staff and parents:
Alderson, P. (1983) *Special Care for Babies in Hospital*. NAWCH, London.
Redshaw, M. *et al* (1985) *Born Too Early*. Oxford University Press, Oxford.

3

SCBU: keeping the baby breathing

Alison J. Stewart, MSc, RHV, RGN, RM
Research Midwife, Bristol Maternity Hospital

Neonatal care has developed in leaps and bounds since 1890 when Pierre Budin opened the first special care baby unit (SCBU) in Paris. In the twentieth century there has been increasing emphasis on reducing the perinatal mortality rate and offering facilities for the care of neonates with increasingly complex problems – particularly those of earlier gestation. There are three types of care for infants needing monitoring or treatment after delivery.

Intensive care   Resuscitative measures and long-term supportive therapy, such as:
• gestation <30 weeks on a ventilator;
• exchange blood transfusion for jaundice;
• major surgery eg, gastroschisis, diaphragmatic hernia.

Special care   An extension of intensive care, babies requiring less supportive measures, such as:
• orojejunal or gastric feeding;
• oxygen therapy eg, headbox and low-flow;
• continuous monitoring of ECG- investigations if apnoeic, bradycardic, or the baby has fits;
• infection screen and treatment with IV fluids and antibiotics;
• terminal care.
   Neonatal unit (NNU) is the term often used to describe one with intensive and special care cots.

Transitional care   Either in a designated ward or in mother-and-baby rooms attached to a NNU where mothers can care for their babies with assistance from staff if necessary, such as:
• babies 34+ weeks' gestation requiring some tube feeds or extra assistance fixing and feeding;
• cleft lip and palate babies;
• babies requiring regular observations eg, diabetic infant or mother or drug addict mother;
• babies from NNU ready for discharge and mothers needing time to get

used to caring for them.

At one time, routine admission policies meant any baby delivered by operative vaginal delivery or caesarean section was admitted to a NNU, but inappropriate referral can cause the parents considerable distress, and contribute to overcrowding and increased staff workload. The trend has now gone in the opposite direction – babies in NNU now tend to be high dependency, and every effort is made to avoid unnecessary admissions – hence the value of transitional care wards where mother and baby are not separated. In the UK approximately 10-30/1,000 neonates need intensive care (Dunn, 1980).

It is preterm babies who have benefited from advances in technology which has led to aggressive treatment methods. Approximately 10/1,000 babies born are under 32 weeks' gestation (Short Report, 1980) and require such treatment as ventilation and enteral feeding. These babies tend to be long-term residents of NNUs, as they progress from intensive care to special care to rooming-in. Very low birthweight babies (VLBW – under 1,500g) have an average stay of over 100 days (Hernandez et al, 1986). Mortality rates vary; Stewart et al (1981) found that 50 per cent with birthweight under 1,000g survived, but it has been argued that the long-term costs in terms of handicap and disability negate the success rate. The same study found 90 per cent of survivors less than 1.5kg appeared normal. Other studies have reported morbidity rates of 25-50 per cent for infants born weighing less than 1,000g (Ovgill et al, 1982; Hernandez et al, 1986; Sandhu et al, 1986).

Low birth weight babies

There are three types of low or very low birth weight babies:

- preterm – born before 37th completed week of gestation, not fully matured, few fat deposits;

- small for gestational age (SGA) – any baby whose birthweight is less than the 10th centile for babies of that gestation;

- combined preterm and SGA.

Table 1 gives a brief list of causes. In general, preterm babies need a high concentration of resources because they are not fully developed and matured and have numerous problems which require treatment.

Whether preterm of not, all neonates have three crucial needs following delivery:

- establishing and maintaining respiration to avoid hypoxia;

- establishing feeding to avoid hypoglycaemia;

- maintaining of temperature.

Babies unable to fulfil these activities need supportive measures.

Causes of premature delivery
• MATERNAL – illness
acute/chronic eg, renal failure,
influenza, pregnancy-induced
hypertension, cervical
incompotence.
• PLACENTAL – infection eg,
rubella.
• FETAL – congenital abnormalities,
multiple gestation.

Causes of SGA
• MATERNAL – illness acute and
chronic (as above).
• PLACENTAL – diminished blood-
flow to the placenta and fetus eg,
after antepartum haemorrhage or
with increased blood pressure or
smoking.
• FETAL – congenital infection,
congenital abnormality, ethnic group
eg, Asians tend to produce smaller
babies in proportion to Western
cultures.

Table 1. Causes of low birthweight.

Respiration

A normal baby begins breathing at delivery in response to physical stimuli, chemoreceptors and respiratory centre stimulation. Once established, a baby of any gestation breathes at a rate of 35-40 breaths a minute. There are a number of signs indicating respiratory distress (which should not be confused with respiratory distress syndrome). These are shown in Table 2. Causes are numerous.

• Tachypnoea <60/min.
• Recession of sternum when
  breathing.
• Cyanosis of skin and mucous
  membranes.
• Grunting on expiration.
• Apnoeas.
• Nasal flaring.

Table 2. Signs of respiratory distress.

Respiratory distress syndrome (RDS)   Insufficient surfactant in lungs to reduce tension between lung surfaces and prevent collapse. Occurs in premature babies, those born to diabetic mothers, or by caeserean section, for example.

Airway obstruction   This could be due to such causes as meconium aspiration at delivery, tracheo-oesophageal fistula or enlarged thyroid.

Pulmonary disease Such as meconium aspiration resulting in chemical pneumonitis.

Infection Pneumonia (congenital or acquired during/post delivery).

Apnoeas Such as prematurity, septicaemia, convulsions, aspiration of feeds, drugs.

	Premature	Term	
PH	7.36–7.45	7.37–7.43	} at 6-24 hours
PO$_2$	8–9.3 kPA	9.3–10 kPA	
PaCO$_2$	4.3–4.5 kPA	4.4–4.8 kPA	} Robertson (1986)

Table 3. Blood gases (these will vary with age and gestation).

The aim of respiratory management is to ensure blood gases remain in a normal range (Table 3). This may involve treating the cause, such as giving antibiotics for infection and/or providing supportive therapy such as some form of O_2 ventilation; head-box or low-flow. With the first two, care needs to be taken to humidify the gases received to avoid a detrimental cooling, drying effect.

Monitoring the effectiveness of O$_2$ therapy
Arterial blood gases These provide information on pH, CO_2, O_2. They are taken either by arterial stab or from an intra-arterial line (radial, umbilical, tibial), which is kept patent by a continuous heparin solution and often attached to a BP transducer to give a read-out. However, there are several dangers in this technique – it is invasive, can be a site for infection, can cause thrombi and occlusion of blood vessels and may lead to fatal haemorrhage if the line becomes disconnected.

Transcutaneous oxygen monitor A probe, with a conductive substance, is attached to the skin, causing localised vasodilation. This provides estimation of capillary O_2, which can be correlated twice daily with arterial gases. It is only a crude measure, since the probe may not be accurately fixed; the skin of preterm babies is friable, while older babies have denser skin. Probes may also measure carbon dioxide levels.

Pulse oximetry A small clasp is secured over a hand or foot and a light passes through the limb to a receptor on the opposite side. An oxygen saturation level of haemoglobin is estimated on the basis of the amount of light absorbed. This is also a crude measure, since it can become dislodged and fail to pick up the pulse, but it is noninvasive and does not adhere directly to the skin.

Ventilation
Ventilation is the mechanical means of inflating the lungs, with options

to control inspired O_2, pressures and rate to achieve normal gases in blood. It is indicated for severe RDS; recurrent apnoeas; abdominal surgery – such as for diaphragmatic hernia or repair of oesophageal atresia; septicaemia; pneunonia and severe meconium aspiration.

There are numerous models, each with different functions, but the types of ventilation include:

- Intermittent positive pressure ventilation (IPPV) – the ventilator does all the breathing.
- Intermittent mandatory ventilation (IMV) – the ventilator provides a certain number of breaths per minute and the baby fills in – used to wean babies off the ventilator.
- Continuous positive airways pressure (CPAP) – the baby does all the breathing but the ventilator keeps a constant low pressure to prevent the lungs collapsing at the end of each breath.

Ventilation can cause a number of complications:
- **Hyperoxia** – retinopathy and retrolental fibroplasia.
- **Hypoxia** – this may lead to brain cell damage and periventricular haemorrhage (PVH) which can in turn give rise to hydrocephalus.
- **Pneumothorax** – with high levels of ventilation or the baby fighting the ventilator.
- **Bronchopulmonary dysplasia (BPD)** from prolonged ventilation.

Care of a ventilated baby
Monitor condition:
– of ventilator and oxygenation: record hourly the rates/pressures/O_2/humidity temperature;

– of baby, colour/are chest movements occurring with ventilator?/ oxygen saturation and response to handling/check lung sounds after movement or suction to ensure endotracheal (ET) tube in place/types of secretion obtained after suction;

– heart rate, attached to ECG, normal 120-160 bpm: tachycardic over 180bpm/bradycardic below 80bpm (varies with individuals and gestation – term babies may have lower normal range) are there any abnormal rhythms or murmurs heard with stethoscope?;

– temperature (axilla, toe, abdominal probe, incubator) alter heat source as needed;

– peripheral circulation if arterial line *in situ*;

– BP, urinalysis, blood sugar every eight hours or as appropriate to detect hypotension and variations in blood sugar level.

Record and report findings, as ventilation settings or concentration of IV fluids may need altering on the basis of this monitoring.

Ensure good ventilation

– ensure the ET tube is' well secured, either taping to the face or tying with tapes to a well-fitting bonnet;
– check X-ray after intubation – the baby should be carefully positioned on his or her back during this procedure without dislodging the tube;
– subsequent careful positioning and movement eg, if weighing;
– suction as needed to remove secretions blocking tube and nose.

This is a sterile procedure using a glove for the tube, and if secretions in the chest are sticky, 0.5ml normal saline may be injected to loosen them prior to suction. Different size suction catheters are available.

– empty tubings of water, which condenses as a result of humidifying, otherwise it will go down the ET tube;
– ensure clothing does not restrict chest expansion;
– orogastric tube *in situ* on free drainage (attached to a mucus extractor) to prevent the stomach being distended by the air blown into it.

Sedation may be necessary to stop the baby fighting the ventilator and trying to breathe out of synchrony. Pancuronium IV will paralyse or a morphine infusion will sedate the baby, but if the ventilator becomes disconnected the baby will not make any respiratory effort, so vigilance must be maintained. The ventilator settings will probably need changing in babies who have been self-ventilating and are now making no respiratory effort, otherwise hypoxia and cyanosis are likely to occur. Current research is attempting to avoid the need to sedate babies by devising a monitor which will enable the baby starting to take a breath to trigger the ventilator to operate in synchrony.

For a variety of reasons it may be necessary to re-intubate a baby, so a spare ET tube cut to the correct length, an introducer, and a laryngoscope should be readily available. There should always be easy access to suction and to a bag and mask with attached oxygen and air supplies.

The incidence of RDS and subsequent complications

Recently the value of surfactant replacement therapy (SRT) has been cited to reduce the incidence of RDS and subsequent complications of bronchopulmonary dysplasia and pneumothoraces (Vaucher *et al*, 1988; Dunn *et al*, 1988). The effects of SRT are still being evaluated and many NNUs are involved in the OSIRIS multicentre trial. Surfactant is manufactured synthetically and supplied as a powder to be reconstituted with preservative-free sterile water. Strict protocols exist in NNUs about the babies for whom surfactant is suitable according to gestation, weight and risk of RDs. Dosage is based on the weight of the child (generally 5ml/kg) and the drug is administered as a bolus slowly into the trachea via a special adapter on the ET tube. SRT may be given at birth and possibly several subsequent doses. Guidelines may exist to delay subsequent ET suction after SRT. The dosage volume can cause a blockage of the airway with decreasing oxygen saturation requiring ventilator peak inspiratory pressure to be temporarily increased to compensate. As with all drugs the infant's condition should be carefully monitored after administration eg, ECG, colour, oxygen saturation, chest expansion and blood gases are sampled to detect post-dosing hyperoxia and hybercarbia.

Positioning   Generally babies are nursed prone to splint the sternum against the mattress and improve lung inflation. The head is turned to alternate sides and, according to unit policy, the neck may be slightly extended by using a neck-roll, such as a rolled up nappy or piece of gauze. As with adults, a change of position is needed at least 4-hourly to avoid damage to tissues, loosen chest secretions, move limbs and muscles and in the case of preterm babies, avoid the skull bones ossifying to produce rectangular, flattened heads.

Temperature   This is likely to be unstable if the baby is in a criticial condition requiring ventilation. Initially the baby may be nursed without clothing and covered with bubble-wrap if this is needed to observe appearance and chest movements. Most ventilated babies are therefore kept in an incubator or heated cot. Incubator care involves carefully regulating the heater controls to ensure a temperature which keeps the baby with a core temperature of 36.6°-36.8°C. Temperature control will be discussed in greater detail in a later chapter.

Feeding   Nutrition is required, but until the baby's condition is stable this will be IV, either dextrose with electrolytes or total parenteral nutrition (TPN). Subsequently feeding may be with milk enterally via either an orojejunal (OJ) or gastric tube. The choice depends on how the baby tolerates the feeds and whether it compromises lung expansion. Feeding will be discussed in more detail in a later article.

Skin and mouth care   Skin damage is easily caused by constantly sticking on probes and monitors and then peeling them off again, as babies do not have the tough skin surface of adults. The skin of preterm babies is particularly friable and may actually peel away with a piece of sticky tape when removed. Mouth care needs to be 2-hourly to moisten the mouth and remove secretions – sterile water on a cotton wool bud is effective. Cord care is needed, cleaning and powdering the cord until it separates. Nappy changing is only required as appropriate to avoid skin damage, such as rashes – this might be every eight hours.

Elimination   This needs to be observed carefully, since critically ill babies may require a diuretic. Urine output can be measured accurately by attaching an adhesive urine bag or by weighing nappies. Any baby who is paralysed with Pancuronium may need bladder expression. This will be discussed in greater detail in a later chapter.

Infection Many respiratory problems are associated with infection, such as group B- haemolytic *streptococcus* which has a high mortality rate. A course of antibiotics such as flucloxacillin or netilmycin may therefore be routinely started until all results of swabs and blood cultures come back as negative.

Drugs Antibiotics may be needed, and premature babies may be prescribed Ethamsylate (capillary stabiliser) for a limited number of doses (16) in prophylaxis against PVH. If apnoeas occur as ventilation is reduced (IMV/CPAP) due to immature respiratory system and not any other cause, a respiratory stimulant may be prescribed, such as Aminophylline. All drugs are given IV until feeds are tolerated.

Minimal handling This means disturbing the baby as little as possible, ensuring all care is in an organised sequence and protecting babies from other professionals who may want to disturb them just when they are having a rest. This is essential for three reasons:
- Sleep is beneficial to any patient and most neonates spend their lives sleeping, in NNU there is little opportunity for this due to the lights, noises and people.
- Any stimulation can alter respiration, even leading to apnoea and bradycardia and that may drop the PaO_2.
- Reduced contact may minimise cross-infection.

Headboxes

These provide an oxygen enriched atmosphere for babies who are managing to breathe of their own accord. If above 50-60 per cent oxygen is needed to maintain a satisfactory PaO_2, this is generally seen as an indication for an alternative method such as CPAP. Attachment to air and O_2 means a given concentration can be regulated. Head boxes are indicated for babies being weaned off a ventilator; those with difficulty with PO_2, such as post-surgery; those with mild RDS or infection.

Observations As with babies on ventilators, when caring for those in headboxes it is necessary to record hourly the oxygen concentration and $TCPO_2$ and then relate it to the baby's condition, probably doing a full set of temperature, heart rate and respirations 2-3 hourly. Otherwise, care is as needed and similar to that for babies on ventilators. It is important to remember that babies in headboxes only receive the specified oxygen concentration if the box has a small hole mainly filled with the baby's shoulders and no other unblocked holes – otherwise the oxygen is lost into the incubator or cot.

As the baby copes in an oxygen level the aim is to slowly reduce it as tolerated until the baby is in humidified air and then ready to try the transition to outside the box. Babies in headboxes are more readily accessible to parents and may be taken out for cuddles, with the oxygen supply maintained via the headbox tubing with just a face mask attached over mouth and nose.

Low-flow oxygen

This is the provision of small amounts of oxygen (measured in cubic centimetres) to a baby who is otherwise thriving and may be discharged home with a portable supply. A small tube (often nasogastric) has the far end sealed and two holes cut and positioned under the nostrils. This is then permanently attached with tape to the cheeks and then connected to tubing going to a piped or portable oxygen supply. It is used in babies with BPD and after ventilation and head-box for those who become cyanosed and distressed if oxygen supplies are totally removed, and need several weeks to be weaned down.

Observations   Rate of flow in relation to respirations and colour should be monitored – $TCPO_2$ may be used intermittently to monitor the baby's response to the concentration. As tolerated, the level is reduced, but if the baby becomes cyanosed or respirations increase, the level may need increasing again. Otherwise the baby is generally in a cot, coping with breast or bottle feeds and may even be cared for and supported at home (Sleath, 1989).

References

Dunn, M.S. *et al* (1988). Two year follow up of infants enrolled in a randomized trial of surfactant replacement therapy for prevention of neonatal respiratory distress syndrome. *Paediatrics*, **82**, 543–7.

Dunn, P.M. (1980) Newborn Care in the UK, in: Short Report 2.244. Second Report from Social Services Commission of Perinatal and Neonatal Mortality. House of Commons, London.

Hernandez, J.A., Offut, J. and Butterfield, L.J. (1986) The cost of care of the less than 1000gm infants. *Clin. Perinatology*, **13**, 461–76.

Ovgill, A.A. *et al* (1982) Early development of infants of 1000gm or less at birth. *Arch. Dis. Child.*, **57**, 11, 823–7.

Roberton, N.R.C. (1986) *A Manual of Neonatal Intensive Care*. Edward Arnold, London.

Sandhu, B. *et al* (1986) Cost of neonatal intensive care for VLBW infants. *Lancet*, **1**, 600–03.

Short Report (1980) Ibid.

Sleath, K. (1989). Breath of Life. *Nursing Times*. **85**, (44), 31–33.

Stewart, A.L., Reynolds, E.O. and Lipscombe, A.P. (1981) Outcome of VLBW; survey of world literature. *Lancet*, **1**, 1038–40.

Vaucher, Y. *et al* (1988). Neurodevelopmental and respiratory outcome in early childhood after human surfactant treatment. *American Journal of Diseases in Children*, **142**, 927–930.

4

SCBU: maintaining the ideal body temperature

Alison J. Stewart, RGN, RM, RHV, MSc
Research Midwife, Bristol Maternity Hospital

As adults, we regulate our body temperature by such methods as taking off or putting on clothing, opening windows, sweating and shivering. Babies are passive and cannot do any of these things, and also have little control over their body responses; for example, they do not shiver in the first few weeks of life unless they are extremely cold (<20°C). They may retain some heat by vasoconstriction, but low birth weight babies (LBW), whether preterm or small for gestational age, have little subcutaneous fat to provide insulation.

Babies may generate heat by thermogenesis in brown fat stores, where the breakdown and reconstitution of triglycerides releases energy which warms the circulating blood, but this method relies on oxygen and glucose, so hypoxic and hypoglycaemic infants are compromised, as are premature infants who do not have large stores of brown fat and have a large surface area/body mass ratio. The easiest way to preserve existing body heat is to stay in a curled up position, but unfortunately, preterm and sick babies tend to lie supine in a 'frog' position, exposing a greater surface area. It is easy for babies to rapidly lose heat by convection, conduction, radiation and evaporation – life can become a grim struggle to offset these effects.

Hypothermia
Reduced PH and PaO_2;
increased O_2 consumption;
recurrent apnoeas;
impaired blood coagulation;
reduced surfactant synthesis in the
   lungs;
fits;
DEATH.

Hyperthermia
Increased fluid loss;
hypernatraemia;
increasing apnoeas;
DEATH.

Table 1. Risks of increased and decreased body temperature.

Every baby has a range known as its neutral thermal environment, which is the 'ideal' at which the baby has to use minimum oxygen and energy to maintain temperature. Normal temperature is axilla 36.5°-37°C, and both high and low body temperatures can have detrimental effects (Table 1).

There are two methods of monitoring babies' temperature:

- thermometer – axilla or rectal;

- probe – abdominal, axilla, toe – there should not be more than a 2°C difference between toe and core – more indicates peripheral shutdown, which may need plasma transfusion to correct it.

Maintaining temperature

General care Certain measures can be taken to minimise cooling effects on babies in general unit just after delivery and in neonatal units (NNUs) in particular:

- Ensure delivery is in a warm, draught-free room, and that the subsequent environment is warm enough.

- Dry all babies at delivery with a prewarmed towel.

- Use appropriate methods to maintain temperature (see below).

- Choose suitable clothing – particularly hats, since the greatest heat loss is from the head.

- Avoid any undue exposure – for example, when nappy changing in a cot, keep the baby's top half covered up.

- Warm all items which come into contact with the baby, such as clothes, water for washing, feeds and gases in ventilators.

- Ensure the baby receives adequate feeding to provide energy to generate heat.

Incubators These provide an enclosed environment which can be regulated by adjusting the heater control. Some will operate on Servo with a probe attached to the infant's skin and linked to the incubator. This will adjust the temperature to achieve a preset infant temperature, and has the advantage of reducing the need to disturb the infant. There is, however, always the danger that with mechanical failure the baby may become pyrexial or hypothermic, and this will only be detected with regular checking of axilla/abdominal temperature.

Variations in weight, gestation, and condition may require considerable differences in environmental temperature needed – for example, at 26 weeks babies need to be 36.5°C and at 34 weeks, 30°C+. Different types of incubators exist with various operating features. The range of temperatures available may vary between a lower range of 29-

35°C for larger, less sick babies and 30-38°C to meet the needs of hypothermic or LBW babies.

Any baby failing to maintain his or her own temperature, and those which are preterm, septicaemic, in shock, post-operation or nursed naked with phototherapy should be kept in an incubator. There are, however, a number of factors to consider in nursing babies in incubators:

- They give limited access in an emergency – some units prefer to use heated cots with overhead heaters.

- Babies are separated from parents by a tangible wall.

- Heat loss, which can be caused by:

Convection – the air current of the circulating fan may be cooling, as may draughts caused by doors opening and closing. If monitoring allows, the baby should be fully clothed, if not, a heatshield with one end closed off can reduce the wind effect.

Radiation – particularly from the incubator if the room temperature is cold, can cool the baby. This means the room the incubator is in needs to be warm. It may also be necessary to cover the baby with bubble-wrap (used in packing parcels) if the baby needs to be nursed naked. Otherwise babies should be dressed in something to provide maximum cover, like an all-in-one Babygro and a hat.

Evaporation – particularly if the baby is immature, since the skin is extremely water permeable. It may be necessary to humidify the incubator to keep the air warm and moist, and possibly wrap the baby in cling-film.

Conduction – which means that anything in contact with the baby must be warm. Normally the baby lies on a sheet on a mattress in the incubator, placing a piece of gamgee underneath the sheet can provide further insulation.

Care of the baby
Careful monitoring of the baby's temperature is essential to avoid under- or overheating. In a hypothermic baby, the aim should be to warm slowly by approximately one degree per hour, as rapid heating or cooling by inadequate regulation of the heating controls can cause babies to develop recurrent apnoeas.

Probes monitoring temperature have the advantage of providing a measurement without disturbing the baby. However, be aware that it may be inaccurate if the baby is lying on the probe or if the probe is becoming dislodged. Probes may be attached to the skin by adhesive tape, but this can cause trauma, particularly to preterm babies, whose skin is friable. Alternatively, a protective pad of stomahesive on the skin, to which probe and adhesive tape are stuck, or securing bandage can be used.

All care such as changing nappies, clothes and sheets should be performed with the baby in the incubator, to ensure minimal exposure to air currents. Gamgee and blankets may be used to protect the baby if procedures require him or her to be exposed with the incubator door down, such as lumbar puncture. Bringing babies out for a cuddle needs to be balanced against whether their condition is stable and whether they will maintain their temperature. Babies of weights such as 700g can maintain their temperature if placed inside their parents' clothing to have the comfort and warmth of skin-to-skin contact (Whitelaw, 1986). Parents need to be taught how to handle and care for their child, for example, by using the port-holes, and also not to see the incubator as a barrier separating them from their baby.

As babies cope with lower temperatures, the incubator controls are turned down, and once they maintain their own temperature at approximately 30°C they are ready to try the transition to a normal cot.

Overhead heater   This provides a radiant heat source which, if small and portable, can be of considerable use when taking a small baby out of an incubator either to change it for a clean one (approximately once a week) or for the baby to be weighed, as it provides an immediate means of keeping the baby warm.

Heated cots   These provide warmth from underneath, and can be regulated to a preset temperature – the maximum generally being 35°C. Heated cots tend to be used with babies who need a little additional warmth but do not require an incubator, and can provide a stepping stone in the transition from an incubator to a normal cot. They are particularly favoured by parents, who find it provides easier access to their child.

Heat shields   A concave piece of perspex, placed over a well-wrapped baby in a cot, can reduce heat loss from convection and radiation. It provides a measure of protection to allow the baby to conserve heat, but does not actually generate heat as the previous methods do. Unless the end is blocked off, for example by covering the bottom with a blanket, however, heat shields act as wind tunnels and actually increase babies' heat loss. Shields are available in different sizes and must be chosen to suit the size of the baby when wrapped in normal coverings. They are especially useful with babies (often preterm 34-36 weeks) who maintain their temperature for most of the time, then drop it when out of the cot feeding, or during the night when the room cools slightly.

Regular monitoring

Whatever method of temperature control is used, the baby's temperature must be checked regularly and appropriate action taken to provide or remove heat on the basis of findings. Teaching parents to be aware of how vulnerable babies can be to heat loss is extremely important, so they can learn, for example, to bath their baby in a warm room with everything ready to hand, to avoid unnecessary delays while the baby is naked. It is probably best not to bath small babies until they weigh 2.5kg or more. The largest percentage of heat escapes from the head, so bonnets can be vital – even if the baby is indoors or in an incubator. Also, bootees and mittens, even over a Babygro, can reduce heat loss from babies' extremities. Several lightweight blankets are more effective than one heavy one, since air is trapped between each layer and provides insulation. Parents need to be able to judge how warm the baby feels, and how to adjust clothing accordingly, both inside and outside the cot or incubator. Underwrapping and overwrapping the baby can both have serious consequences, and parents whose baby has been in the tropical environment of a NNU may have difficulty and be worried about 'getting it right' at home. Teaching them how to control their baby's temperature is a vital part of discharge preparation if they are to be able to maintain their baby at the correct temperature competently and confidently.

Reference
Whitelaw, A. (1986) Skin to skin contact in the care of very low birth weight babies. *Maternal and Child Health*, 11, 7, 242–46.

Bibliography
Roberton, N.R.C. (1986) *A Manual of Neonatal Intensive Care*. Edward Arnold, London. A helpful and very detailed text.

5

Adequate intake to allow optimum development: feeding and elimination in SCBU

Alison J. Stewart, RGN, RM, RHV, MSc
Research Midwife, Bristol Maternity Hospital

Adequate caloric and fluid intake is necessary for survival. The energy requirements of neonates are approximately 120-150kcal/kg/day, with between 60-180ml/kg/day in the first week of life. Breast milk is obviously the first choice where practicable, as it is ideally suited to human requirements, but artificial milks are now modified to resemble breast milk as far as possible. By providing nutrition for growth and development, a feeding regime avoids hypoglycaemia, which, if prolonged below 1mmol/l may contribute to brain damage. However, there are a number of factors to consider in feeding preterm babies.

Physical problems

Poor glycogen stores and sometimes immature gastrointestinal tracts of very low birth weight (VLBW) babies mean they are particularly at risk – especially of hypoglycaemia – and preterm babies have a small capacity stomach with a lax cardiac sphincter, so feeds may easily be regurgitated. Bowel peristalsis may be variable in preterm babies, sometimes causing delay and distension, and they may need assistance to pass stools. At less than 34 weeks' gestation, most babies tend to have a poorly developed suck and swallow reflex. It is also important to remember that a small stomach filled to capacity can cause respiratory embarrassment.

Methods for providing adequate nutrition include:
- IV fluids – dextrose and electrolytes;
- total parenteral nutrition (TPN);
- enteral feeding – gastric or jejunal;
- oral feeding by breast or bottle. (See Figure 1).

The choice of feeding method will depend on the baby's condition – with all babies requiring treatment or close monitoring, it is essential to calculate feeds/fluids to ensure there is adequate intake. The amount depends on the baby's gestation, and either birthweight or current weight (whichever is larger). It also takes into account factors like cardiac failure or phototherapy to either restrict or increase intake.

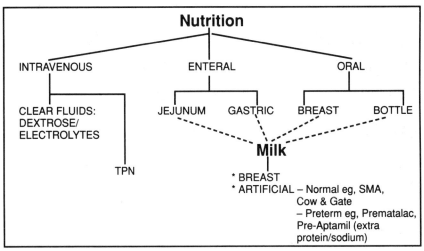

Figure 1. Options for feeding a baby.

Intravenous feeding
Indications:
- respiratory disorders;
- prematurity;
- septicaemia;
- abnormalities/infection of the gut, such as meconium ileus or necrotising enterocolitis;
- immediately post-surgery;
- prolonged hypoglycaemia which does not respond to milk feeds.

Site Veins used are generally peripheral (arms, legs or scalp), though they may be central veins if a line is inserted during surgery.

Solution This can be a dextrose solution alone, such as 10 per cent, or a dextrose solution with electrolytes, or TPN comprising Vamin amino acid solution with glucose, electrolytes and water soluble vitamins, and lipid fat emulsion.

Care
- To prevent infection, the line must be changed every 24 hours, and strict asepsis maintained when making solutions and attaching lines.
- The IV site should be checked regularly for infection or tissuing – babies cannot complain of pain. As most solutions are irritant, necrosis can occur if there is leakage into the tissues.
- A volumetric infusion pump is generally used to ensure infusion of the correct amount of fluid, as these provide a readout of hourly rate, total

amount to date and pressures at cannula – which, if rising, may indicate fluid leakage into the tissues.
• Mouth care must be maintained, since the baby is taking nothing orally.

Observations   The baby's growth should be checked by weighing daily or alternate days – rapid gain may indicate cardiac failure. Fluid balance between intake and output must be watched, and urinalysis and BM-Stix checked eight hourly. Preterm babies have an intolerance to sugar, so glycosuria and hyperglycaemia may occur, requiring a reduced level of dextrose in the solution. Specific gravity of urine of over 1015-1020 can indicate dehydration. Blood pressure must be taken eight hourly, as hypotension may suggest hypovolaemia.

Enteral feeding

Naso-/oro-jejunal (NJ/OJ)   A small silastic tube (different size lumens are available) is passed from the mouth or nose to the jejunum. This takes approximately eight hours to advance through the stomach, and needs to be checked to ensure it is *in situ* before commencing feeds. This is done either by X-ray or by passing water down a nasogastric (NG) tube. If the water is not obtained up the OJ tube, it is probably *in situ*. The tube is attached to a syringe pump for continuous infusion of milk at a set rate per hour, and is kept in place either by taping it to the baby's cheek or if it is an oral tube, by use of an individually produced dental plate with a groove into which the tube slots.

Indications   Babies (generally preterm) who are unable to tolerate gastric feeding, for example because it causes respiratory embarrassment and apnoeas, are often given NJ or OJ feeding. The method is also often used for babies whose condition has stabilised and are on a ventilator.

Care   The baby should be nursed prone, otherwise there is the risk of aspiration if feed is regurgitated. Milk must be changed four to six hourly to avoid bacterial growth in the heat of the NNU, and an orogastric (OG) or NG tube should be kept *in situ*, aspirated four hourly and left on free drainage. This provides a check on regurgitation of milk through the pylorus or the tube moving back into the stomach. Feeds should be stopped if there is abdominal distension, recurrent apnoeas or vomits. The baby's mouth should be moistened and cleaned regularly with cotton wool buds and, if a dental plate is used it must be removed and cleaned twice daily.

Observations   These include the amount of aspirates – if small they should be replaced down the jejunal tube, but if large, the position of the jejunal tube should be considered – it may need advancing further. Response to feeds should be monitored for vomiting, apnoeas and stool consistency, to indicate how well the baby is tolerating and digesting feeds. A check should be kept on the baby's weight – if it is static or decreasing, the method of feeding or the milk used may be inappropriate.

Orogastric or nasogastric (OG/NG)   A tube is inserted from mouth or nose to stomach – again, different size lumens are available. The tube's position can be checked by aspiration and testing the liquid's acidity with litmus paper, or by injecting air into the stomach and listening with a stethoscope. NG and OG feeding are generally used to provide bolus feeds rather than continuous feeding, and the decision to pass orally rather than nasally is based on the size and gestation of the baby – babies are compulsory nose-breathers and if a small nostril would be totally occluded by a tube, it should be passed orally.

Indications   The methods are useful in VLBW babies, who are generally without respiratory problems, and have poor or absent suck reflex. Babies failing to complete feeds may also benefit – those of 34 weeks' or less gestation often tire easily, and a tube and breast regime may help until they have the energy to take all their feed by breast or bottle. Tube feeding can also be used with babies who have mechanical difficulties – for example, cleft lip and palate babies may have difficulty sucking until a plate is fitted.

Care and observations   The baby should be nursed prone, as for jejunal feeding, and before each feed it should be checked that the tube is *in situ* and not dislodged. The daily amount of feed can be calculated into manageable portions – for example, small babies may tolerate small feeds two hourly while larger ones may prefer them three hourly. The tube should be aspirated prior to giving a feed to ascertain that it is being absorbed, and feeds should be stopped if there is abdominal distension, recurrent apnoeas or vomiting. Mouth care is as for jejunal feeding.

Transition of feeding regimes

There may be considerable variation between units as to when one method is used as opposed to another, but generally there should be a progression towards oral feeding as the baby improves. Once the baby shows interest in sucking, one OG feed daily can be replaced by a breast or bottle feed, and as these are tolerated, further ones can be introduced. The skill is in changing regime and assessing the baby as an individual and to avoid stressing or tiring him or her by trying to achieve too quick a conversion to all breast or bottle.

Oral feeding, whether by breast or bottle, requires fixing, sucking and completing a feed with sufficient calories and fluid in a reasonable time. If the baby tires or fails to complete feeds, one feed time merges into the next.

Supplements and weight gain

Many VLBW babies have insufficient stores of vitamins and iron laid down *in utero*. It is generally recommended that babies weighing less than 2.5kg or of less than 36 weeks' gestation have vitamins A, C and D and iron supplements daily to promote growth and prevent late onset anaemia. Iron supplements may be discontinued by the time the baby is a year old if haemoglobin levels are satisfactory.

Weight gain is a good indication that the baby is getting adequate nutrition and also of clinical wellbeing. Normal babies tend to lose up to 10 per cent of their birthweight in the first week and then regain it by the end of the second week, subsequently gaining about 200g per week. Small or ill babies may gain weight very slowly unless there is fluid retention and oedema, while those on TPN show an increase once the lipid is added. Generally babies are weighed on alternate days unless there are indications for daily weighing, such as renal failure.

Elimination

A normal infant tends to pass 25-60ml urine/kg/24 hours. In comparison to adults, babies have a restricted ability to regulate fluids and electrolytes, and particularly if they are sick or preterm, they may end up with an imbalance. For example, hypernatraemia can develop with the evaporative water losses under phototherapy. In critically ill babies, urine output needs to be monitored carefully, either by weighing nappies or measuring the quantity collected in a bag stuck to the genital area.

Meconium – a thick, greenish-black substance which is formed of mucus, dead epithelial cells and bile pigment in the gut *in utero* – is normally passed within 24 hours of delivery, and indicates that the lower gastrointestinal tract is patent. Subsequently, stools become yellow once feeding is established. Stools are softer in breast-fed babies than in those who are bottle-fed, since there is less residue after absorption. Frequency of stools can vary considerably from four or five times daily to once every four days, but if there is delayed passage with considerable distension, there may be obstruction, infection or constipation, occasionally needing suppositories. Offensive stools can indicate infection, and loose green stools may be due to infection or under- or over-feeding. Blood or mucus in the stools needs rapid investigation since it may be necrotising enterocolitis and this can be fatal if not treated.

Neonates must be closely monitored for their response to feeds or IV fluids. There may be only small indications the baby is not coping or behaving as expected, and findings need to be placed in the context of the baby's clinical condition, weight and elimination pattern.

Bibliography
Roberton , N.R.C. (1986) *A Manual of Neonatal Intensive Care*. Edward Arnold, London.
A helpful and very detailed text.

6

A cry for help? Management of postoperative pain and discomfort in neonates

Paul Cornick, RGN

Post Registration RSCN Student, Queen Elizabeth School of Nursing, Birmingham

Many medical and nursing textbooks, when dealing with the care of neonates, make little or no reference to pain and analgesia. In recent years the topic of neonatal pain has attracted more attention. This chapter examines this topic, and looks at measures that can be taken to minimise discomfort following neonatal surgery.

Can neonates feel pain?

The physiology of neonates differs from that of older infants and children: they have higher circulating endorphin levels, and also immature pain conducting pathways and receptor systems (Hatch, 1987). They do however have the necessary anatomy required for, and capability of, feeling pain (Anand and Hickey, 1987). Pain thresholds, and the reaction to pain by neonates may differ, but an ability to feel pain is present. The immaturity of neonatal nervous systems has led to a traditional belief that they either cannot feel pain or cannot distinguish noxious fron non-noxious stimuli.

Many people now feel, on observing neonates during medical procedures, that it is readily apparent they can feel pain. It has been shown that they mount a stress response to surgery (Anand et al, 1985) and that this is reduced by perioperative analagesia (Gauntlett, 1987). A questionnaire sent to paediatric anaesthetists has recently revealed that 80 per cent of respondents believed neonates can feel pain (Purcell-Jones et al, 1988) and it has been said that the burden of proof is now with those who believe neonates cannot feel pain (Owens, 1984).

Recognising the pain

If we accept that neonates may feel pain, we must look first at how to recognise it and then how to minimise it following surgery. Clinical staff have no definite criteria or guidelines for assessing presence or degree of pain. They must use their knowledge and experience to determine if it is present or if other factors explain the behaviour and condition of a baby.

Pain can affect stability and clinical condition in several ways; altering respiratory pattern and rate, heart rate, blood pressure and arterial oxygen saturation (Hatch, 1987; Yaster, 1987). Some types of body movement, facial expression and crying can indicate pain (Owens, 1984; Anand and Hickey 1987). There has been a report of severe pain caused by glaucoma inducing a 'sleeping fit' in an infant (Burton and Derbyshire, 1958), but there have been no reports of this reaction occurring widely or following surgery. To interpret calm sleeping postoperative neonates as being in pain would be wrong and potentially dangerous if powerful analgesics were then administered. Abnormal withdrawal and quietness however may, in this context, be caused by pain.

Nursing interventions

Many neonates cope very well following surgery. For these babies attentive and thoughtful nursing is sufficient to maintain comfort. Nursing staff can aid comfort with the use of oral toilet, comforters, sheepskin bedding and bean bags. Keeping babies dry and warm and minimising handling, noise and bright lights will also help. If medically feasible, maintenance of good hydration and early oral feeds may also aid the neonate's comfort.

One small study has suggested that stroking, for comforting purposes, of neonates during painful nursing procedures can have the opposite effect to that desired, and actually increase distress (Beaver, 1987). These procedures (eg, suctioning and repositioning) should be performed as quickly as possible, with rest given between them.

Some neonates do not settle or cope well after surgery. If it is felt that a baby is in pain, or may be in pain, it would seem reasonable to give some form of analgesia after the above measures have failed to provide comfort. There are several different approaches to neonatal analgesia. Powerful analgesics are rarely necessary and two drugs, paracetamol and codeine phosphate are often adequate.

Use of paracetamol

Paracetamol is effective in relieving peripheral pain. It works by inhibiting prostaglandin synthesis. Pain fibres are stimulated by the local production of prostaglandin, during the inflammatory process, at the site of injury. Little has been published about the use of paracetamol in neonates and its effectiveness is not agreed upon. Some centres use it with apparent success, and a dose of 10mg/kg has been noted by one centre as being effective – often after a single dose.

Paracetamol is only recommended by the Committee on Review of Medicines for use in patients over three months of age. However, the manufacturers know of no clinical reason for this, and encountered no problems prior to the recommendation (Owen, 1988). Paracetamol is safe to use in non-jaundiced neonates (Booker, 1987), but caution is required with repeated doses as the neonatal liver is very immature.

Administration and absorption of paracetamol can be affected by gastrointestinal tract surgery. If a baby's condition will allow, paracetamol can be given orally or rectally, whichever route is further from the surgical site. Problems may then be minimised. Rectal paracetamol does, however, present the problem of dividing suppositories to obtain small doses.

Use of opioids

Codeine phosphate is an opioid drug. The opioids work by acting on the central nervous system and by modifying the response to nerve signals induced by painful stimuli. This means they may be more appropriate for visceral or severe pain.

Codeine phosphate is not widely used in neonates, but is thought to be both safe and effective. A dose of 1mg/kg is reported as working well and causing few problems, none when used as a single dose medication (Purcell-Jones et al, 1987). Other, more powerful, opioids are also used for neonatal analgesia, such as morphine, pethidine, papaveratum and fentanyl, and their use with spontaneously breathing neonates is perhaps the most controversial area of this topic.

There have been many reports of respiratory depression caused by opioid analgesia (Hatch, 1987) and it must be appreciated that there is a high degree of risk (Gauntlett, 1987). Papaveratum is perhaps the most dangerous of these opioids, as it is not a pure or single drug and its effects are thus more unpredictable. Pethidine was, in the past, thought safer than morphine (Way et al, 1964) but a recent study reports the reverse (Purcell-Jones et al, 1987).

Those who advocate the use of powerful opioids in non-ventilated neonates suggest it is safe in an intensive care setting (Gauntlett, 1987; Purcell-Jones et al, 1987). Any neonate given opioids requires constant supervision ('one-to-one' or 'one-to-two') and close monitoring. Respiratory side effects can then be noted and action taken. Apnoea monitors can be useful but should not replace close observation. Medical expertise and facilities for ventilation must be available.

Infusion of opioids is thought to be safer than bolus doses (Gauntlett, 1987; Hatch, 1987; Purcell-Jones et al, 1987) and fentanyl is suggested by some to be a more effective drug than morphine for infusion.

Use of ventilation

Opioids are commonly used in ventilated neonates. Elective ventilation following major or difficult surgery can be combined with opioid infusion to provide safe, powerful analgesia, and modern ventilation methods mean this should not prove hazardous (Gauntlett, 1987). A neonate treated in this way can be kept pain free and well rested, allowing healing to commence with a minimum of strain being put on delicate surgical repairs. The unpredictable length of time that large opioid doses take to clear in neonates (Koren et al, 1985) make close supervision necessary to ensure safety following extubation.

Local anaesthesia

Local or regional nerve blocks and/or local infiltration are an alternative way of providing analgesia. They work by blocking noxious stimuli at source and preventing conduction in nerve fibres. This form of analgesia is thought to be safe (Yaster, 1987). Nerve blocks can be used in the operating theatre for perioperative and postoperative analgesia. Infiltration of wound sites with local anaesthetic solution can be carried out both during surgery and postoperatively.

The most commonly used drug for this type of analgesia in neonates is bupivacaine solution up to a maximum dose of 2mg/kg. The most serious complication of bupivacaine is convulsions caused by accumulated dosage or overdosage. Another possible complication is introduction of infection through use of wound infiltration. Highly selective choice of sites, for example away from rectal or genital areas, would perhaps minimise this risk. The use of nerve blocks or the infiltration of local anaesthetic solution can reduce the need to consider other forms of analgesia with more potentially serious side effects.

Reye's syndrome

One form of pain relief not yet discussed is the use of nonsteroidal anti-inflammatory drugs (NSAIDS). These can provide strong analgesia without respiratory side effects. Unfortunately their use is strongly contraindicated in neonates. There are two reasons for this. First, there are problems in accurately obtaining small doses. Second, is the association of these drugs, particularly aspirin, with Reye's syndrome.

Use of sedation

There can be a need to aid the comfort of surgical neonates who are not thought to be in pain, but are agitated and unsettled for other reasons. Examples are babies who are maintained nil by mouth for long periods following surgery, or who are distressed by ventilation. Sedation can have a role in the care of such babies, but it is important to note that if sedation, without analgesia, is given to a neonate suffering postoperative or other pain, the result may be increased excitement rather than sedation (Roberts, 1984). Two drugs used for sedation in this type of situation are chloral hydrate and triclofos sodium; of these, chloral hydrate is the better documented and more widely used (Franck, 1987). Their action is similar, but triclofos is less of a gastric irritant.

In conclusion, it appears that neonates are capable of feeling pain and discomfort. Minimising this, if done safely, must surely benefit the babies, their parents and the staff working with them.

A neonate cannot tell us he or she is in pain, and no clear guidelines are available for assessing this – further study and research are very much needed. In the meantime, staff must use their clinical skills and experience to judge which type of intervention is most appropriate.

Thoughtful and skilled nursing care appears to be important and beneficial. If pharmacological intervention is used, several approaches are available, and the choice of which type of analgesia, drug and route of administration to use can be made in the context of individual clinical situations. The main influence on such decisions must be safety.

Neonates are different from other patient groups, and staff must ensure they are treating a neonate in pain rather than their own adult perception of pain. It would be immoral to leave babies needlessly in pain, but also immoral to place them in danger through unsafe or inappropriate use of analgesics. Our aim must surely, and simply, be to help our youngest and smallest patients as much as we can without placing them in danger.

References

Analand K.J.S., Brown, M.J., Causon, R.C. et al (1985) Can the human neonate mount an endocrine and metabolic response to surgery? *Jnl of Pediatric Surgery*, **20**, 1, 41–84.

Anand, K.J.S. and Hickey, P.R. (1987). Pain and its effects in the human neonate and fetus. *New England Journal Of Medicine*, **19**, 317, 21, 1321–29.

Beaver, P.K. (1987) Premature infants' response to touch and pain: can nurses make a difference? *Neonatal Network*, **6**, 3, 13–17.

Booker, P.D. (1987) Postoperative analgesia for neonates? *Anaesthesia*, **42**, 4, 343–44.

Burton, I.F. and Derbyshire, A.J. (1958) Sleeping fit caused by excruciating pain in an infant. *American Journal Of Diseases of Children*, **96**, 258–60.

Franck, L.S. (1987) A national survey of the assessment and treatment of pain and agitation in the neonatal intensive care unit. *Jnl. Obst. Cynae. and Neonatal Nursing*, **16**, 6, 287–93.

Gauntlett, I.S. (1987) Analgesia in the neonate. *Brit. Jnl. Hosp. Medicine*, 518–19.

Hatch, D.J. (1987) Analgesia in the neonate. *British Medical Journal*, **294**, 920.

Koren, G., Butt, W., Chinyonga, H. et al (1985) Postoperative morphine infusion in newborn infants: assessment of disposition characteristics and safety. *The Journal of Pediatrics*, **107**, 6, 963–67.

Owens, M.E. (1984) Pain in infancy: conceptual and methodological issues. *Pain*, **20**, 213–30.

Purcell-Jones, G., Dorman, F., Summer, E. (1987) The use of opioids in neonates. *Anaesthesia*, **42**, 12, 1316–20.

Purcell-Jones, G., Dorman, F., Summer, E. (1988) Paediatric anaesthetists' perceptions of neonatal and infant pain. *Pain*, **33**, 2, 181–87.

Roberts, R.J. (1984) Drug Therapy In Infants: Pharmacology Principles And Clinical Experience. W B Saunders, Philadelphia.

Way, W.I., Costley, E.C., Leong Way, E. (1964) Respiratory sensitivity of the newborn infant to meperidine and morphine. *Clin. Pharm and Therapeutics*, **6**, 4, 454–61.

Yaster, M. (1987) Analgesia and anaesthesia in neonates. *The Journal of Pediatrics*, **111**, 3, 394–95.

Bibliography

Anand, K.J.S. and Hickey, P.R. (1987). Pain and its effects in the human neonate and fetus. *New England Journal Of Medicine*, **19**, 317, 21, 1321–29.

This paper looks in detail at the requirements for pain perception.

Franck, L.S. (1987) A national survey of the assessment and treatment of pain and agitation in the neonatal intensive care unit. *Jnl. Obst. Cynae. and Neonatal Nursing*, **16**, 6, 287–93.

This survey examines beliefs about and treatment given for neonatal pain.

Owens, M.E. (1984) Pain in infancy: conceptual and methodological issues. *Pain*, **20**, 213–30.

This paper applies the concept of pain to infants and examines methods of studying and recognising pain in them.

Purcell-Jones, G., Dorman, F., Summer, E. (1987) The use of opioids in neonates. *Anaesthesia*, **42**, 12, 1316–20.

This study examines administration of opioid analgesia to postoperative neonates.

Purcell-Jones, G., Dorman, F., Summer, E. (1988) Paediatric anaesthetists' perceptions of neonatal and infant pain. *Pain*, **33**, 2, 181–87.
This survey of anaesthetists reveals that although belief in neonatal pain perception is widespread, use of analgesia is not.

Acknowledgements
Grateful thanks to the many medical and nursing staff who gave comment, criticism, advice and encouragement during the writing of this paper.

7

Time to hand over the baby: parental care of the preterm infant

Suzanne Hazell, BA, RGN
Neonatal Unit Sister, Llandough Hospital, South Glamorgan

Parents usually embark on parenthood anticipating a normal baby, to be born vaginally at 40 weeks' gestation. While most prospective parents think of handicap as a vague possibility, few consider that of a preterm delivery of 10 or more weeks. If a premature delivery is anticipated however, a visit by one or both parents to the neonatal unit (NNU) will help familiarise them with the new surroundings and technology, and meeting some of the NNU staff. Being able to see babies of similar gestation who are progressing well will help reduce the shock of seeing their own baby in intensive care for the first time. If such a visit is not possible, a visit by a member of NNU staff for a chat on the ante natal ward can be helpful.

After the birth of a preterm baby, the parents may only glimpse their baby being resuscitated and are unlikely to be able to touch him or her until later in the NNU. It is usually the father who is first able to visit the unit, by which time the baby will be ventilated, monitored with ECG, PO_2, PCO_2 and temperature probes and will have peripheral intravenous (IV) and, possibly, arterial lines. Total care is provided by NNU staff, and parents are usually left frightened and bewildered - most have had no prior experience of a NNU or known any other parents of extremely preterm babies. NNU staff must help parents come to terms with their new baby during these first visits to the unit, so that they can eventually take over the complete care of their baby.

Supporting the parents

Once the baby has arrived in the NNU, the parents will need a great deal of support and information to help them accept their baby, who they are unable to cuddle or show easily to other members of the family and friends. Staff can help by showing they understand the parents' feelings, and by emphasising the baby and not just the surrounding technology. Richards (1983) observed it takes much longer for parents to 'get to know' their special care baby compared with parents of well babies, and it has been suggested that prolonged separation increases the risk of future child abuse (Lynch and Roberts, 1977). The study sample of Lynch and Roberts was small and many other factors can influence abuse of children, factors which also predispose premature birth.

There are many ways these problems can be eased: a photograph taken as soon as possible after the baby is admitted to the NNU should be given to the mother, who may not be able to visit her baby for several hours, and parents should be assured they can take their own photographs. Family centred care is also important in a NNU and should be extended to include the wider family and friends - parents should be able to bring visitors to see their baby and be able to tell them how he or she is progressing. Siblings need to be able to visit their new brother or sister, and may like to put a small present in the incubator. Making the unit look less clinical also helps reduce parental stress: pictures, wallpaper or colourful friezes help, as does dressing the baby in pretty clothes. Here again, family and friends can participate by making small items such as bonnets, bootees or a small blanket. NAWCH (1985) noted that making units appear more homely and less clinical was becoming common among NNUs, and several units have regular ongoing formal and informal parent groups which can help parents cope with the situation (Boukydis, 1982).

Helping parents care for their baby

Introducing parents to the practical tasks of care in the unit and the intricacies of the technology involved is the first step to education of parental care, and parents are much more likely to accept the situation if they understand what is being done and why. A visit by a member of NNU staff to the mother on the postnatal ward can be reassuring if she is unable to see her baby for a few hours after delivery.

Many unfamiliar concepts and terms will have to be learnt by parents while their baby is in the unit and as parents are unable to assimilate all the information given during early visits, many NNUs produce small booklets for parents, which should be given with reassurances that anything that is not understood can be re-explained or enlarged upon. When parents visit the unit, they should be given repeat explanations of the baby's condition and the monitors used, as they may still be too overwhelmed to know what to ask - once the nurse starts talking, parents often respond with their questions and worries. A more detailed book is available for parents who desire it (Kitchen et al, 1983), and there is also a small book suitable for siblings (Althea, 1986).

Staff new to NNUs usually care for well babies first, gradually progressing to the high dependency area, thus building up their skill, knowledge and confidence. For parents, the dilemma is suddenly finding themselves dealing with an intensive care situation without having had any practical or emotional preparation. NNU staff can usually remember some aspects of their first days in the unit and the apprehension they felt caring for 'their' first ventilated baby, and they must now appreciate how parents will feel for their own baby. Parents are, initially, unwilling to do anything for fear of disturbing the wires and setting off alarms, often saying that staff are better at handling sick infants, and so deterring themselves from wishing to participate in care. With help, however, they can begin with simple activities such as touching, stroking and talking to the baby, and it is important at this stage that staff stress the baby's need for love and comfort from his or her mother and close family, and the importance of touch and sound of their voices.

Having been shown how to avoid dislodging any of the equipment, parents can carry out mouth care, washing and nappy changing. They should be shown how to gently clean inside the baby's mouth around the ET tube using a cotton bud dipped in sterile water, and, if the lips become dry in the incubator atmosphere, to apply a small amount of liquid paraffin to them using a cotton bud. Nappy changing ceases to be such a daunting task after a few attempts and mothers will be surprised at the smallness of the preterm size nappies, which will be too large for the very smallest babies and need to be cut in order to fit.

Nutrition is an important part of the baby's welfare and, even though introduction of milk feeds may be delayed, mothers can be encouraged to express their milk for when the baby commences enteral nutrition, breast milk being a gentle introduction to gut function. They should be given all the information they need to help them collect their milk, with the use of the breast pump and the need for cleanliness clearly explained. The milk is then put into sterile bottles provided by the hospital and labelled with the name, date and time of collection, and can be frozen for up to three months and used within that time if oral feeds begin. Mothers often comment that this is one of the few important tasks they can carry out for their babies in the first days following birth.

Sharing mutual experiences

The early days of an infant's life may be fraught with setbacks such as jaundice, pneumothorax, infections, anaemia, apnoeas, bradycardia, tachycardia and frequent resiting of IV lines, and each condition must be explained to the parents if and when it arises. One means of helping parents realise that they and their baby are not unique is to show them short case histories of other babies who have had similar experiences - those compiled with photographs will show a baby's progress with a more personal touch. Introducing parents to other people whose baby has been in the NNU enables them to discuss their worries with others who have had similar experiences. Parents gradually take over more of their baby's care as the ventilator and monitors are removed. They can breast, bottle or tube feed their baby, give physiotherapy and medicines (such as vitamins and supplements), which will be given at home.

Preparing for discharge

A wide range of nursing tasks can be taught to parents. Paul, as the following case history shows, was born at 27 weeks to a mother of three young children, and after several weeks ventilation developed bronchopulmonary displasia (BPD), a chronic lung condition which can take many months for a baby to outgrow. Paul became oxygen dependent, needing four-hourly physiotherapy and suction as well as a 'cocktail' of drugs for several more weeks after discontinuing ventilation. The baby's parents lived nearly an hour's journey from the hospital, and were only able to visit him once or twice weekly, with the rest of the family visiting less often. It became evident that Paul could be taken home with all the necessary equipment, and this was quickly accepted by his parents who introduced the idea to their three other children, who were allowed to look after and hold him. Paul and his family were prepared for his discharge from hospital in the following ways:

- The physiotherapist came to teach Paul's parents how to carry out chest physiotherapy and oropharyngeal suction and two suckers were prepared for home, one battery and the other electrically operated.
- Oxygen therapy had to be continued, and Paul's parents were taught how to monitor the oxygen concentration and to refill and change the small portable cylinders light enough to take on the pram. These procedures were taught by the porters. Lengths of tubing were extended from the oxygen cylinder to a blind-ended tube, making the baby and his oxygen supply more manoeuvrable. A nasogastric tube with a tight knot in the end was used and two small holes were cut in the side of the tube at the same distance apart as the nostrils and the tube was then taped to the baby's cheeks.
- Paul needed restricted fluids because of some degree of heart failure resulting from the BPD, and Calloreen was added to his normal milk to meet the required amount of nutrition. The volume was to be no more than 180mls/Kg, and his mother was to be taught how to calculate this; some of this volume was to be added to his solids.
- The drugs prescribed for Paul were: multivitamin, iron, potassium chloride, cotrimoxazole, aminophylline and frusemide. A 24-hour timetable was devised with times (to coincide with feed times), drugs and dosages. Drugs were obtained in easily calculable volumes and marked syringes for the aminophylline and frusemide.

To help prepare Paul's mother adjust to caring for him at home, she spent three nights in the area attached to the NNU. During this time she took over complete care of Paul, and had the opportunity to discuss any problems which had not arisen during her previous short visits. She also visited the children's ward to meet some of the nursing staff, as it was likely that Paul would need future hospitalisation, being prone to chest infections as a result of BPD. This approach combines family-centred care (McHaffie, 1987) with multidisciplinary teaching.

It is impractical to expect parents to take over much of the care in the high dependency area of a NNU, as most are unwilling to do so, but as the baby improves and progresses, they can do more. Although most babies continue to improve and are discharged home with no more than vitamin and iron supplements and a few follow-up appointments, some remain in the medium dependency category for several months. On discharge, it is important to allay parents' fears that their baby is not really ready to go home, and to give them more confidence (McHaffie, 1987). Follow-up appointments will be frequent, possibly weekly at first, but as slow progress is maintained, fewer visits to the clinic are required and less medical equipment is needed at home. Even babies like Paul eventually need no more added oxygen, physiotherapy, fewer drugs and less controlled fluid intake and can be treated like a normal baby.

References

Althea, (1986) *Special Care Baby*, Dinasaur Publications, Collins, Glasgow.

Boukydis, C.F.Z. (1982) Support groups for parents with premature infants in NICUs. In: Marshall, M., Dasman, C., Cape, L., *Coping With Caring for Sick Newborns*. W.B. Saunders, Philadelphia.

Davis, J., Richards, M., Roberton, N. (1983) *Parent-Baby Attachment in Premature Infants*. Croom Helm Ltd, Beckenham.

Kitchen, W.H., Ryan, M.M., Richards, A.L., Lissenden, J.V. (1983) *Premature Babies – A Guide for Parents*. Thorsons, Melbourne, Australia.

Lynch, M. and Roberts, J. (1977) Predicting child abuse: signs of bonding failure in a maternity unit. *British Medical Journal*, 1, 3, 624–26.

McHaffie, H. (1987) Caring for very low birth weight babies. *Midwives Chronical*, 100, 1198, supplement xiv-vi.

Thornes, R. (1985) Parent participation. Results of a NAWCH survey. *Nursing Mirror*, **27**, 160, 20.

Handout: if your baby is in a neonatal unit

Welcome to the neonatal unit (NNU). This handout tells you about your baby and the procedures which may be carried out on him or her.

After the birth
You will be upset at being separated from your baby so soon after birth, and anxious for his or her wellbeing in the NNU. If your baby was born prematurely (preterm), he or she will seem small and vulnerable in the incubator and surrounded by medical equipment. The doctors and nurses will explain what is happening and what all the monitors are for. They will also show you how to care for your baby, so you can help, even if you feel nervous at first. Whenever you want any information, even if you have been told before, ask when you next visit the unit. You will learn an enormous amount about your baby but will not be able to remember it all at once.

Visiting
- Parents may visit at any time, day and night.
- You may telephone at any time.
- The direct line number is ....
- Brothers and sisters may visit, but no other children, while relatives and friends may visit, two at a time accompanied by you.

Preterm babies
Preterm babies have large heads and tummies and rather thin arms and legs. This is normal – they look more in proportion by the time they were due to be born. Some also have soft hair on their body, but this disappears gradually.

Feeding your baby
If you wish to breastfeed, you should start expressing your breasts as soon as possible – the ward staff will show you how. If your baby cannot take milk yet, and is being fed through a vein, your milk can be frozen until the baby is ready for it. If you do not wish to breastfeed your baby at home, you can still express milk for when he or she is either very poorly or very small if you wish, or you can choose from the milk formulas already in the unit. Preterm babies usually begin taking milk via a tube passed through the nose into the stomach until they can suck from the breast or bottle.

Getting better

As soon as your baby is well enough, he or she can come out of the incubator for a cuddle, firstly with Mum and Dad, then when he's better with other relatives. You will see other babies in the unit getting better and going home – some stay just a few days and others many weeks if they are born extremely early. As your baby gets better, he or she will be able to wear clothes – you can bring some in if you wish, and take them home to wash. If you put your baby's name on them, there is less chance of them getting lost if they get washed with the unit's baby clothes.

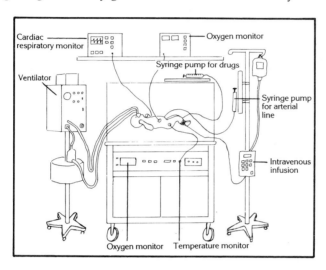

As babies' conditions improve, they may be moved around the unit. We may have to do this without letting you know if, for example, a new baby comes in or your baby does not need intensive care anymore, so don't worry if you can't find your baby – just ask a nurse. While your baby is improving, you will gradually take over more of the care when you visit.

Getting ready for home

By now you will have been shown how to do everything you need to do for your baby at home, such as bathing, breastfeeding or making up feeds. Babies are normally allowed home when they weigh about five pounds, are feeding well without tubes, and their general condition is good. To help you feel more confident, you and the baby's father (if he wishes) can stay in the mother's room for a night or two, caring for the baby as if you were at home, so you get used to caring for your baby day and night while you can still ask for help.

Home at last

Your baby has been used to a warm NNU and you may need to keep the house warmer than usual for the first few days. Once your baby has adjusted he or she will be comfortable in a room in a temperature between 16–20°C. Babies can get too hot and with young babies it is better to use blankets as bedding since a layer can be added or removed according to how warm your baby feels. Older babies, over one year old, can have a duvet since they can wriggle out of it if they get too hot. Remember when you go outside your baby will need more clothes than you, including a bonnet, since he or she can easily get cold sitting in a pram in the wind.

Babies develop from the time of conception so if your baby was born early you should expect him or her to do things at the appropriate time after his or her due date, not the date when he or she was actually born. For example, born in December and due in April, your baby should be sitting in October-time (6 months after April). In fact, because your baby was born early he or she has had more opportunity to practice so is likely to do it earlier than many babies born in April.

You will probably have an appointment to bring your baby back to a clinic for check-ups, and this is when you will be told how he or she is progressing. Once your baby is home, if something is worrying you, do not hesitate to ring the unit. They may still be able to help or say whether your own doctor should deal with it. Remember, it is important that your baby has a good start in life after being sick in NNU, so he or she needs to have immunisations for protection from future illness.

We have your baby soon settles down at home, and will bring you a lot of happiness. The unit staff love to hear how babies are getting on so, if you have a few minutes after your clinic appointment or you are passing by, drop in and see us again.

Family Support in Caring

8

Weaning: a first step to independence

Elizabeth M. Horne, MA
Publishing Director, Professional Nurse

Myra Ibbotson, PhD, BSc, SRD
Freelance Nutritionist and Dietitian

Weaning, the gradual transition made by babies from a diet comprised largely of milk, to one which is more diverse and predominantly solid can be a stressful time for both baby and parents. Cultural and social backgrounds lead to a range of varying parental expectations and beliefs about the process, and can lead to controversy over its ideal timing and planning. Nurses and health visitors can do much to help parents wean their babies with as little stress as possible for both parents and child by giving appropriate advice and allaying unnecessary worries.

Psychological aspects
The intake of a good balance of different nutrients is essential for normal growth and development during childhood and for health throughout our lives. Perhaps because it is such a basic requirement for life, feeding is a powerfully emotive activity and can cause parents considerable anxiety if problems arise along their baby's route to a healthy 'normal' diet. Parents - and particularly breastfeeding mothers - see the weaning process as representing and illustrating the changes in the relationship between the adult and the growing child: from complete dependence as a newborn baby to the relative independence of the child (Lowen, 1980). Small children attach associations to new foods and flavours which may strongly influence their food preferences later in life and the new foods encountered during the weaning process set important precedents for the future.

The confidence and competence with which a mother approaches the feeding of her baby depend on the advice she gets when the baby is routinely checked and weighed. Insufficient advice can leave her uncertain and nervous, and these feelings will be picked up by the baby. *Absolute* weight gain, measured against one of the standard growth charts, is not as important as a pattern of steady weight gain and a clearly healthy baby (even if the baby weighs less for its age than the average) - babies (and adults) vary considerably in the body weight which is 'normal' for them. If parents are made to feel they are underfeeding the baby, their concern and loss of confidence can actually lead to feeding problems as mealtimes become emotionally charged events instead of what is ideally a fairly uneventful part of the normal routine.

When should weaning begin?

There are no strict rules as to when weaning should start, and as with so many developments, children vary considerably in their requirements and the speed at which these change. Unless there are special medical reasons, however, no baby should be offered solid foods before the age of four months, and most babies will certainly need solid foods by the time they reach 14lbs (6.5kg). Babies have a store of iron at birth which lasts four to six months, and weaning should take place at this age to avoid anaemia. New tastes of solid foods should be introduced ahead of the baby's need for these foods. Even for a very small baby, whose weight will not reach 14lbs for several weeks, it is advisable to start introducing tiny tastes when he or she is seven or eight months old. If this is left too late, the child will find the new flavours and feeding methods less easy to accept.

First solid foods

Tiny quantities (1-2 teaspoons) of solid foods should be given at each feed to start with, accompanied by the usual amount of milk. Rice mixed with expressed breast milk or formula milk or other gluten free cereals should be given at first, with the gradual introduction of new flavours. 'Solid' foods should be semi-liquid in texture: lumps or pips may cause choking if swallowed. Parents should never force new food on their baby - it is important that they respect the definite preferences he or she shows.

   At first, solid foods are only needed for the extra calories they provide - protein, fats, vitamins and minerals are all supplied from milk. *Any bland food,* so long as it is liquidised or mashed, will provide these extra calories: potato or carrots mashed with milk or stewed and puréed fruit (avoiding those with pips, such as gooseberries) are good examples. Baby rice and cereals are often chosen as the first solid foods because they are rich in iron, while their bland, milky flavour makes them more acceptable to the baby than many other foods. Salt should not be added to babies' food as it can strain their kidneys, while spices and exotic seasonings can burn the mouth or irritate the digestive system. Too much fat or sugar will also upset babies' digestion.

   Commercially available cans and jars of baby food with their limited lifespan provide more food than a baby is willing to accept in the early stages of weaning, and can only be kept refrigerated for 24 hours. The unused contents should be decanted into lidded containers for storage and any surplus thrown away after 24 hours. Dehydrated foods are more useful at this stage because they can be used gradually.

The recent reports of contamination of baby foods with glass splinters and other foreign bodies have caused manufacturers to encase their jars in tamper-proof plastic sleeves. Parents should check this seal is intact before buying jars. Foods packaged in boxes are less liable to interference since they cannot be easily resealed.

The other recent scare which may affect babies is that of salmonella in eggs, and at the time of going to press, the Department of Health has recommended that babies and children should not be given raw or partially cooked eggs. However they are prepared, eggs should be cooked until both the yolk and white are solid.

It takes some time for babies to adapt to using a spoon instead of sucking. Offering a teaspoonful of solid food part way through a feed of milk will help the baby adjust. If a small spoon is used and held just between the lips, the baby will be able to suck the food far enough back in the mouth to swallow.

Solids as meals

Babies show that they need more solid food by wanting to start a meal with solids or refusing more milk after they have been given solids. Enthusiasm for solid food may vary from day to day, and is important that parents let their baby take the lead - food should be enjoyed. Allowing babies to play with food and eating 'finger foods' such as a raw carrot, crust or rusk will encourage enjoyment and can help babies learn to handle food for themselves. It is vital, however, that babies are always attended to when eating, to ensure they do not choke - they only learn to move food from the front to the back of the mouth at five months.

An important element of babies' early feeding is the comfort they derive from sucking. During weaning they learn new skills of feeding from spoons and drinking from cups, but still require the comfort of sucking, especially at bedtime and perhaps at the first feed in the morning. Most children give this up naturally around the time of their first birthday.

How much food?

A six month old baby needs, on average, about 800 calories per day. These are mostly obtained from milk, which also provides all the protein, fats, minerals and vitamins required, but as milk consumption drops, foods which provide calories, iron and vitamins A, D and C should be introduced. A pint of milk alone will provide enough protein, calcium and B group vitamins for babies' needs. Commercially available 'high protein' foods have no extra benefit, and nor do meat or fish, while skimmed milk does not have sufficient nutrients and should not be given to children under five, and semi-skimmed milk to children under two.

Which foods?

There is very little which adults normally eat which babies cannot tolerate, although salt, hot spices, alcohol, coffee and tea should be avoided. All food must, of course, be in semi-liquid form and presented in tiny quantities. Ready-prepared baby cereals are valuable foods fortified with iron and vitamins, and are easy to use. Cans or jars of baby food, however, tend to provide less concentrated nutrients than the equivalent home-cooked versions. Babies from families with a strong family history of allergies or atopic disease should avoid potentially allergenic foods such as cow's milk (goat's milk is a less allergenic substitute) and fruits, eggs and wheat until they are at least six months old.

It is very important for parents to feel confident and in control of this stage in their baby's development - fears which are not addressed promptly will lead to problems later on. Parents should be encouraged to contact their health visitor or GP if they feel the need to discuss developments in their child's feeding patterns.

References
Lowen, A. (1980) *Fear of Life*. Macmillan Publishing Company, New York.
Department of Health. (1988) Press release 88/445.

9

Planning for the best start in life: a guide to infant feeding

Susan Holmes, PhD, BSc, SRN, FRSH
Lecturer, Division of Nursing Studies, University of Surrey

Although trends in infant feeding are continually changing, its interpersonal aspects remain constant and, from birth, feeding is closely linked to emotions (Howard, 1984). For example, infants make their need for food known by crying and displaying physical signs such as restlessness and sucking; maternal responses result not only in the provision of food but also of warmth and comfort. Thus the apparently simple act of meeting the biological need for food becomes linked to emotional satisfaction and helps promote mother-child bonding.

Feeding is also of great importance to the future development of the child and may exert a significant influence on adult health. It is not, therefore, surprising that the DHSS (1988) has noted increasing interest in infant feeding/nutrition. It is worth noting, however, that although current dietary guidelines advocate reduced intakes of fat and saturated fatty acids and moderate intakes of simple sugars and salt, infants are specifically excluded from these guidelines (DHSS, 1984), and the National Advisory Committee on Nutrition Education has warned of the dangers inherent in modifying a child's diet on the basis of recommendations directed at adults (NACNE, 1983). Since infants' energy needs are high, the recommendations on dietary fat have been modified for children under five years of age (DHSS, 1988).

Growth and development

Infants grow rapidly during the first year of life. During the first three months, they gain an average of 25–95g per day, which slows to 15-21 g per day during the next three months (Fomon, 1982). Over the first year body weight triples, brain weight doubles and length (height) increases by 50 per cent (Rohr and Lothian, 1984). Such intense growth requires considerable nutritional support.

During this period, normal infants respond to the need for food by crying and by oral reflex responses which initiate sucking, swallowing and biting movements. Initially, sucking and swallowing function as a 'chain reaction', since swallowing can occur only after the sucking reflex is initiated (Howard, 1984). Biting (rhythmical opening and closing of the jaws) is due to stimulation of the gums and, until three to five months, is a simple reflex action preceding the development of a true chewing pattern. The gag reflex, which is present from birth, becomes weaker once chewing mechanisms have developed (Mueller, 1972).

Swallowing is facilitated as the suck-swallow reflex fades and control of head and neck movements improves (Holmes, 1987). At the same time, hand-mouth and eye-hand coordination develop and the child begins to sit unaided, becoming more able to participate actively in the feeding process. As independence in feeding increases, however, so does the desire for autonomy, and children often play with their food and utensils and become vocal during meals. Such behaviour does not necessarily signify food rejection, but represents exploration and the beginning of the development of independence.

Weaning, therefore, represents the first stage in the development of independence and is a time when infants begin to learn new motor skills and become used to a variety of new tastes and textures of food, not all of which will be acceptable - transitory feeding problems are, therefore, likely (Holmes, 1987).

Physiological factors

Although the gastrointestinal (GI) tract has developed to the point at which digestion and absorption can occur, its development continues for some time until complete maturity is reached. For example, it is common for regurgitation of ingested food to continue until about 15 months, when oesophageal maturation should be complete (Winter, 1984), while absorption of glucose is somewhat limited in the first year compared with adults (Younoszai, 1974). Similarly, the availability of pancreatic enzymes is restricted (Klumpp and Neale, 1930) and, when combined with a limited secretion of bile, this means fat absorption is not as efficient as in adults. This is particularly true when fat is derived from cow's milk, when 5-20 per cent is excreted; breast-fed infants, in contrast, excrete less than 7 per cent of ingested fat (Winter, 1984). Protein digestion, however, appears to reach normal levels in both term and pre-term infants (Borgstrom, 1960).

Nutrient needs

Because growth is so rapid during the first year, infants have high nutrient needs, making infancy a time of great nutritional vulnerability. Nevertheless, it must be remembered that children, like adults, have individual needs, and while dietary guidelines and recommended dietary allowances (RDA) are available (DHSS, 1979), they are intended as guidelines for evaluating the nutritional adequacy of the food consumed by populations, rather than individuals. Thus, dietary recommendations must not be applied indiscriminately, but should take account of individual needs.

Energy (calorie) intake   As infancy is the period of life when weight gain is most rapid, a high energy intake is necessary; during their first six months, infants need an average of 115kcal/kg body weight/day. At one year of age this decreases to approximately 105kcal/kg. This must be supplied by breast milk or formula feeds.

As in all diets, energy is derived from carbohydrate (CHO) (4kcal/g), fat (9kcal/g) and protein (4kcal/g). Both breast milk and most formula feeds provide approximately 70kcal/100ml, of which 40-50 per cent are CHO, 11 per cent protein and 50-55 per cent fat (DHSS, 1988).

Protein requirements　These depend on both body size and the rate of growth. During infancy the demands of rapid growth mean that protein requirements are high to allow formation and maturation of body tissues. Indeed, at this time, the need for amino acids greatly exceeds that of adults and, during the first six months, the RDA for protein is 2.5/kg/body weight/day, equivalent to a minimum intake of 1.8 protein per 100kcal. Breast milk provides less total protein than unmodified cow's milk, although it is both readily digestible and of high biological value. The high protein content of cow's milk results in an unacceptable renal solute load, so that unmodified milk should not be given to infants. Breast milk also provides other non-protein substances which may be beneficial in promoting growth (Lawrence, 1980).

Fat　Serving various functions in an infant's diet, fats supply a major proportion of the total energy and provide fat soluble vitamins (A, D, E, and K) and essential fatty acids (linoleic and linolenic acids). In general, the fat in breast milk is different from that in milk derived from other mammals and is also better absorbed (Harries, 1982). For this reason, all or part of the butter fat in formulae based on cow's milk is removed and replaced by mixtures of animal and vegetable fats so that the fatty acid composition more closely approximates that of breast milk; this also leads to more complete absorption.

Carbohydrates　The major carbohydrate present in both human and animal milk is lactose which, when digested, yields a mixture of glucose and galactose. Glucose is an essential energy source and galactose is necessary for the synthesis of the glycoproteins and glycolipids essential to the central nervous system (CNS).

Vitamins and minerals　Milk from a well-nourished mother normally provides all the vitamins, minerals and trace elements essential for a healthy infant, so the vitamin content of feeding formulae should match that of human milk (Scott and Bishop, 1985). However, although most infants are unlikely to become vitamin deficient, some - particularly those breast-fed by a mother in poor vitamin status - may be vulnerable so that supplementary vitamins are recommended from the age of one month until at least two years of age and, preferably, until the age of five (DHSS, 1988).

Food intolerance

Despite the inevitable variations between children, general dietary principles can be applied and guidelines for 'healthy feeding' have been proposed (DHSS, 1988) Breastfeeding is actively recommended during the first few months of an infant's life (WHO, 1977; DHSS, 1988), because the nutritional and immunological properties of breast milk obtained from women in good health provide a complete food designed specifically to support and protect human infants.

Immunoglobulins, particularly IgG, are actively transported across the placenta, so infants are born with adequate stores. Nonetheless, neonates are susceptible to infection because the immunological system is immature. Colustrum and breast milk are, therefore, important sources of additional immunoglobulins and breastfeeding is believed to protect infants against a variety of illnesses (Chandra, 1978; 1979).

While, in theory, the antibodies in breast milk may protect infants by absorbing antigenic proteins, the evidence on which this is based is equivocal (DHSS, 1988). Chandra (1979), for example, has suggested that breastfeeding decreases the incidence of atopic eczema, while others (Kramer and Moroz, 1981) have found no difference in incidence between breast-fed and formula-fed infants. The Royal College of Physicians (RCP, 1984) have described asthma, eczema, rhinitis and GI disturbances as clinical manifestations of infantile allergic reactions to food and, at times, GI symptoms may result in a life-threatening failure to thrive. The college concludes that, although food allergy may be a significant problem in affected infants, its true incidence is unknown. In rare instances, some infants are intolerant of substances present in breast milk, which causes such reactions as vomiting or colic. Such intolerance is believed to be triggered by a maternally-ingested protein excreted in the milk (Gerrard, 1979; Cant *et al*, 1986), but the clinical implications of maternal transfer and the benefits of maternal dietary exclusion have not yet been convincingly demonstrated (DHSS, 1988).

Formula feeds may be suitable alternatives for infants with intolerance or for those whose mothers are unable or unwilling to breastfeed. Such formulae are manufactured specifically to replace human milk, and are designed to provide the sole source of nutrients for bottle-fed infants (Fomon *et al*, 1979; Mettler, 1982; Wharton, 1984). Most formulae are based on cow's milk, although some contain other proteins such as soya protein; these are usually reserved for infants with special requirements, such as those known to be intolerant to cow's milk.

Although such formulae are nutritionally adequate they do not confer anti-infective or immunological protection, which is why breastfeeding is actively recommended. Breastfeeding also has other advantages - for example, it may help to develop closeness between mother and child, although some women may resent it for restricting their lifestyle. In practical terms, it is less expensive and less time consuming than buying and mixing formulae and washing and sterilising bottles, and so simplifies 'feeding on demand'. Bottle-feeding may, however, free mothers to work outside the home and also encourage others (such as the father) to accept at least some responsibility for feeding.

Most formulae are powders simply requiring the addition of water and, provided mixing instructions are followed, will satisfy all the infant's needs. If a bottle-fed infant appears to be hungry the amount of each feed and/or the number of feeds given in the day may be increased, but the concentration of the feed should *not* be increased (DHSS, 1988).

Weaning

Weaning is the stage when children must become accustomed to the loss of mother's milk which is gradually replaced with semi-solid food. It usually occurs between four to six months, when infants are physiologically able to assimilate solids, sufficient pancreatic enzymes are available, the kidneys can tolerate increased solute loads and the intestine is less permeable to foreign proteins (Holmes, 1987). Weaning does not begin at the same age for all infants, however, and the exact timing varies according to both local custom and individual preference - some infants may wean themselves early.

Although milk remains a dietary staple, further additions can be made as follows: strained, enriched cereals (preferably wholegrain), strained fruit, cooked, strained vegetables and meats and, at seven to nine months, finely chopped meat. It is important to remember that the child is now developing food habits: firmness combined with patience and encouragement to try new flavours and textures, will favour the development of sound eating habits. By about nine months, the child should be eating the foods consumed by the rest of the family, albeit in smaller amounts.

There are two challenges to face in weaning: foods added to the diet must maintain nutritional status, and the psychological impact of the transition from liquids to solids must be eased as much as possible. Weaning is critical in development as infants face many new demands as they become increasingly independent and learn to talk, walk and eat solid foods. Parents too may face difficulties in adjusting since, although they may be proud of their child's achievements, they may also feel rejected, particularly if the child has weaned itself early. Mothers must be reassured that weaning is a natural development and that they still have important functions - weaning is an interactive process, and mothers must use their resources both to identify and prepare appropriate and acceptable foods. They must also replace other functions previously served by breast or bottle; for example, feeding may provide a means of comforting a restless baby and may induce sleep, so alternative approaches must be identified. Similarly, parents often feel that if their child does not eat well, they are failures as parents, but children often sense their parents' anxiety and respond by refusing food. Weaning is therefore, a period of change and feeding often becomes one of the major areas of conflict (Brazelton *et al*, 1984).

Feeding toddlers and preschool children remains challenging. The goals remain the provision of adequate nutrients required to support growth and increasing levels of physical activity, and to continue the development of appropriate food habits.

By the age of one year, nutritional needs can be met by a daily diet including three to four glasses of milk, two small servings (two to three tablespoonsful) of meat or egg, two of cereal, two of fruit and one of vegetables. As age increases, milk remains important and a variety of foods will ensure an adequate nutrient supply. Quantity may, however, become increasingly important as growth slows and appetite decreases. Forcing food onto a child may be counterproductive - most will consume adequate amounts, provided their appetite is not dulled by between-meal snacks. As children begin to accept more foods, portion size can be increased and additional portions given.

It can be seen that the nutritional needs of infants are high if normal growth and development are to occur. Satisfactory feeding can be achieved using breast or bottle although, in the latter, care must be taken to ensure that mixing instructions are closely followed. In both cases vitamin supplementation is recommended (DHSS, 1988).

Appropriate feeding will contribute to the development of a healthy child and will help to promote mother-child bonding, forming the basis of a relationship which will continue into adult life.

References

Borgstrom, B. (1960) Concentration and absorption of protein and glucose in duodenum of premature infants, *Am. J. Dis. Child.*, **99**, 338–42.

Brazelton, T.B. *et al* (1984) Developmental feeding issues. In: Howard, R.B. and Winter, H.S. (Eds) Nutrition and Feeding of Infants and Toddlers. Little, Brown and Company, Boston.

Cant, A.J. *et al* (1986) Effect of maternal dietary exclusion on breast-fed infants with eczema: two controlled trials. *BMJ*, **293**, 231–33.

Chandra, R.K. (1978). Immunological aspects of human milk. *Nutrition Revue*, **36**, 265–85.

Chandra, R.K. (1979) Prospective studies of the effects of breastfeeding on incidence of infection. *Acta. Pediatr. Scand.*, **68**, 691–94.

DHSS (1979) Recommended Amounts of Energy and Nutrients for Groups of People in the United Kingdom. Reports on Health and Social Subjects, No 15, HMSO, London.

DHSS (1984) Diet and Cardiovascular Disease. Reports on Health and Social Subjects, No 28. HMSO, London.

DHSS (1988) Present Day Practice in Infant Feeding: Third Report. Reports on Health and Social Subjects, No 32. HMSO, London.

Fomon, S.J. (1982) Body composition of reference children from birth to age ten years. *Am. J. Clinical Nutrition*, **35**, (Supplement), 1169–73.

Fomon, S.J. *et al* (1979) Recommendations for feeding infants. *Pediatrics*, **63**, 52–59.

Gerrard, I.W. (1979) Allergy in breast-fed babies to ingredients in breast milk. *Ann. Allergy*, **42**, 69–71.

Harries, J.T. (1982) Fat absorption in the newborn. *Acta. Pediatr. Scand.*, **299**, (Supplement), 17–23.

Holmes, S. (1987) The young vegetarian. *Nursing Times*, **83**, 51–55.

Howard, R.B. (1984) The infant feeding experience. In: Howard, R.B. and Winter, H.S. (Eds) Ibid.

Klumpp, T.G. and Neale, A.V. (1930) The gastric and duodenal contents of normal infants and children. *Am. J. Dis. Child*, **40**, 1215–18.

Kramer, M.S, and Moroz, B. (1981) Do breastfeeding and delayed introduction of solid foods protect against subsequent atopic eczema? *J. Pediatrics*, **98**, 546–68.

Lawrence, R.A. (1980) Breast Feeding: A Guide for the Medical Profession. C V Mosby, St Louis.

Mettler, A.E. (1982) Infant formula. *Acta. Pediatr. Scand.*, **299**, (Supplement), 58–76.

Mueller, H. (1972) Facilitating, feeding and prespeech. In: Pearson, P. and Williams, C. (Eds) Physical Therapy in the Developmental Disabilities. Charles C. Thomas, Springfield.

NACNE (1983) A Discussion Paper on Guidelines for Nutrition Education in Britain. Health Education Council, London. Rohr, F.J. and Lothian, J.A. (1984) Feeding throughout the first year of life. In: Howard, R.B. and Winter, H.S. (Eds) Ibid.

RCP (1984) Food Intolerance and Food Aversion. Royal College of Physicians, London.

Scott, K.J. and Bishop, D.R. (1985) Nutrient content of milk products: water soluble vitamins in baby milk formula. *J. Diary Res*, **52**, 521–28.

Wharton, B.A. (1986) Food for the weaning: the next priority in infant nutrition. *Acta. Pediatr. Scand.*, **323**, (Supplement), 96–102.

Winter, H.S. (1984) Development of the gastrointestinal tract. In: Howard, R.B. and Winter, H.S. (Eds) Ibid.

WHO (1977) 27th World Assembly: Part one, Infant Nutrition and Breast Feeding. Official Records of the World Health Organisation, **217**, 20–47.

Younoszai, M.K. (1974) Jejunal absorption of hexose in infants and adults. *Junior Pediatrics*, **85**, 446–49.

10

Silent nights

Marjorie Keys, RGN, HVCert, DipHV
Health Visitor, Cupar, Fife

The idea of 'good sleeping patterns' is obviously subjective – what one parent considers to be a good pattern may be unacceptable to another. Similarly, the term 'sleeping problem' is difficult to define, as it depends entirely on the parents' perception of the situation – they must decide for themselves if a problem exists for them. Perhaps a good sleeping pattern is best described as one which fits in with the customs and needs of the rest of the family and avoids disruption of the parents' sleep during the night.

Studies have shown that sleeping difficulties are one of the commonest problems experienced by parents of young children. John and Elizabeth Newson (1965) found, in a study of 700 one-year-olds in Nottingham, that 35 per cent of mothers had been woken by their babies on the night before the interview. Interviewing mothers of four-year-old children, they found that 20 per cent still woke at night, some only once or twice a week, but some much more frequently (Newson and Newson, 1970). In 1968, Seiler, a Scottish GP set out to examine the prevalence of sleep problems in children aged between six months and five years. He found that in his survey of 234 children, 40 per cent had been a sleep problem at some time.

In my own health visiting practice, a close examination of visits during a recent typical four-week period, shows that sleeping disturbances are a frequently mentioned problem. During this period, sleeping difficulties were expressed at over one third of my visits (see Table 1).

	Age		
	0 – 1	*1 – 5*	*Total*
Total child/visits	38	35	73
Problem*:-			
Sleeping*	16	11	27
Feeding*	11	4	15
General Health*	9	5	14
Behaviour	0	6	6

*Problem indicates difficulty expressed, however slight. Parents were asked specifically about each of these topics. Two children in a household counted as two visits. Where more than one problem mentioned, recorded in all relevant columns.

Table 1. Visits to families with children under five years in a four week period.

Sleep cycles and their relevance

Since research into sleep first started in 1952, a standard language for describing different levels of sleep has evolved, and sleep is said to have two forms – orthodox and rapid eye movement (REM) 'dreaming' sleep. Orthodox sleep has four stages, from light sleep which is easily roused to almost total oblivion. Adults spend about 80 per cent of their time in deep sleep but babies less, and we all go through the four stages of sleep several times each night. One full sleep cycle, known as the ultradian rhythm, takes about 100 minutes in adults, but only about 50 minutes in infants (Haslam, 1984).

Babies, like the rest of us, are most prone to wakening during stage 1 sleep. If a baby then requires the help of a parent to get back to sleep, parents may be disturbed several times a night and are likely to be often woken from deep sleep.

Effects on the parent

The effects on the rest of the family can be insidious and near-catastrophic. A baby or child with a 'sleeping problem' will almost always catch up on the required sleep the next day, but for many parents this is impossible. Although studies may show that adults can survive on remarkably little sleep (Horne, 1981), an exhausted mother who has no expectation of ever getting enough sleep can find life unbearable. She becomes short-tempered with the whole family, has no energy for anything but the most basic tasks, loses interest in her marriage and in outside activities and often loses self-esteem, particularly if she feels the sleeping problem is her fault. Worst of all, the resentment felt towards her baby in the middle of the night can spill over into the daytime hours, and she may indeed begin to hate her child more than she loves him.

Parents in this situation often resort to giving the wakeful child literally anything he demands in the middle of the night, so that they can all get some sleep. Babies may be given several bottles of milk a night; toddlers brought downstairs to play in the early hours of the morning; children allowed to force parents out of their own bed. Often, parents are unaware that other families are suffering a similar fate and feel ashamed of their inability to cope. Surprisingly often they do not ask for help and during my own visits I have found there is sometimes no disclosure of sleeping problems until the parents are specifically asked how their child sleeps at night. They may then describe the most appalling difficulties which have hitherto gone unmentioned.

A problem solved?

Helping parents who are suffering from disturbed sleep can be a great challenge. Some are so desperate they will agree to try almost anything, while others may be afraid of making a bad situation even worse. Sometimes there seems no reason for the wakefulness, and all that may be appropriate is help for the parent to cope with the sleeping pattern, rather than change it. Occasionally avoidance of dietary stimulants such as food additives and caffeine may make a difference. In the vast majority of cases however, what must be suggested is a change in the parents' responses, and a health visitor must exercise enormous tact if she is to help parents realise that they can alter the situation without making them feel that it has all been their fault in the first place.

Several excellent books on helping children to sleep well are available, (eg Douglas and Richman, 1984; Haslam, 1984), but often a parent will not turn to these until a problem has become established. By educating parents in appropriate ways of responding to their children during the night, and by using the handout, which can be given to parents before their babies reach the age at which they can 'waken at will', good sleeping patterns can often be established by the parents' efforts alone. This has two major benefits:

- By knowing how to avert problems, difficulties are less likely to occur, the parent is less dependent on professionals for advice, and self-esteem is enhanced.

- The methods advocated are based on the principle of responding to children in a consistent way and parents also learn to avoid unwittingly giving 'rewards' for undesirable behaviour. The skills thus learned are easily applied to other aspects of parenting and can be used to advantage in a variety of situations.

References

Douglas, J. and Richman, N. (1984) *My Child Won't Sleep*. Penguin, London.

Haslam, D. (1984) *Sleepless Children*. Futura, London.

Horne, J. (1981) Why we need to sleep. *New Scientist*, November, 429–431.

Newson, J. and Newson E. (1965) *Patterns of Infant Care in an Urban Community*. Pelican, London.

Newson, J. and Newson, E. (1970) *Four Years Old in an Urban Community*, Pelican, London.

Seiler, E.R. (1968) Sleep Patterns in Children. *Practitioner*, **208**, 271–276.

Handout: getting your baby to sleep at night

Some parents, either through good luck or good management, find that from the age of about three months their children sleep throughout the night, every night, settling happily at bedtime and waking full of energy in the morning. If this does not sound like your family, you are not alone – studies have shown that about *one third* of one-year-old babies have disrupted sleep patterns, and that means an awful lot of tired parents!

While there are certainly ways you might cope with regular night-time disturbances once they have become established, many parents feel that they could avoid a lot of stress if they were able to help their children develop acceptable sleep patterns as babies. This handout shows how this might be done.

Sleep – what is it?

First, we have to know something of the nature of sleep. Sleep is essential to us all, but while some adults cope happily with five hours per night, most children require much more, and babies most of all. The 'average' baby of nine months might require about 14 hours sleep out of 24; perhaps such a baby would sleep from 7.30pm to 6.30am, then have an hour's sleep in the morning and another nap in the afternoon.

If we look more closely at the sleep between 7.30pm and 6.30am we would see that she does not have the same depth of sleep throughout, but that in common with the rest of us, she alternates between very deep sleep, when she would be difficult to rouse, and periods of lighter sleep when at times she is almost awake, and indeed is certain to waken if disturbed. The speed with which she then goes back to sleep depends very much on how she has learnt to settle.

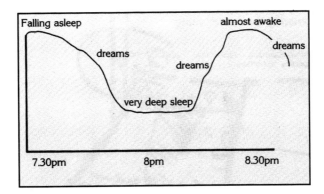

What happens when your baby falls asleep. This kind of 'sleep cycle' will be repeated many times during the night.

Settling methods

Settling babies to sleep in the first few weeks of life becomes something of an endurance test for many parents. Most will adopt almost any method which works at the time, and this can include bottle or breast-feeding, giving a dummy, swaddling, rocking, patting, singing, encouraging thumb-sucking and taking for rides in the car.

While any of these methods may be ideal for very young babies, those of five or six months and older can very quickly become dependent on one method of settling to the exclusion of all others. The result of this is that not only is the rocking or feeding necessary at bedtime, but it becomes necessary several times a night during the baby's 'almost awake' period.

If the normal settling method is not then immediately available, the baby is aware that something is missing; she will not fall asleep without her required settling method because she does not know how to, and she is very likely to protest! An important factor begins to emerge here:

If your baby requires your help for her preferred settling method, you will be disturbed every time she needs to get back to sleep.

Since she may be 'almost awake' seven or eight times a night, that can mean a lot of disturbance – so, what can you do?

The sucking connection

Little babies often like to suck until they are asleep, and will often fall asleep while feeding. If your baby is still doing this at six to seven months of age, it could be time to gently help your baby learn how to settle alone. This means regularly and consistently putting your baby in her cot at sleeping times *still awake*, but, does not necessarily mean that you must deprive her of breast or bottle, which can be offered equally well on awakening rather than on going to sleep. Alternatively, you can continue to give these at bedtime, providing that you do not let your baby fall asleep while still sucking.

It also does not mean that you will suffer a screaming baby for weeks on end because, with consistent behaviour on your part, your baby should learn her new routine well within a week. In this case, when your baby cries in her cot, at bedtime or during the night, you should go to her regularly to reassure her calmly, but *do not give the settling method* as a means of getting her to fall asleep. It is important that you do not offer any other settling method such as singing or rocking which requires your involvement in its place. You should find that after the first few nights your baby will quickly learn how to settle alone. She will continue to have several 'almost awake' spells every night, but will settle to sleep again if undisturbed, and will only cry persistently if in discomfort or pain.

The attention-seeker

Perhaps your baby is a little older and has proved herself capable of falling asleep without your assistance, but is beginning to show signs of wakefulness during the night. Sometimes you might feel that there is no reason for her to deliberately stay awake; you begin to get the feeling that she is 'playing you up'. From the baby's point of view, the explanation is simple:–

It is much more fun to see mum and dad several times a night than to lie alone in a cot – even if they do get exceedingly cross!

The wakening habit can therefore become something of an attention-seeking routine, especially with babies of 10 months and more. When this results in repeated screaming for attention throughout the night, once again a consistent response on your part can pay dividends.

Be a bore!

Go to your baby when she cries, calmly tell her that it is time to go to sleep. Tuck her in if you wish, but keep verbal and physical contact to a minimum and leave the room quietly. Do not plead with her, sing to her, play with her, smack her or shout at her in an attempt to get some silence, as any of these responses can be more interesting (and rewarding) for your baby than going back to sleep. Simply repeat the above procedure every five or 10 minutes and remember your aim is to be as *boring as possible*!

The first and second night you try these tactics, you could find yourself getting out of bed up to 20 times, but for most parents the long-term benefits outweigh the short-term discomforts. By the fifth night you should see remarkable progress; unless your baby is most exceptionally determined, she will have realised that there is simply no point in making a fuss.

Can you help your baby to sleep well?
Try to:
- Establish a relaxed and predictable bedtime routine.
- Provide a comfortable sleeping environment.
- Put baby down for the night when sleepy but not overtired.
- Put baby in cot awake, both at bedtime and for daytime naps.
- Help baby learn to settle alone, without assistance (a baby with a dummy may require assistance if it keeps getting lost).
- Attend promptly to cries during the night but keep interaction brief; be as 'boring' as possible.
- Avoid giving any 'reward' for crying (eg singing, rocking) that your baby may wish you to repeat.
- Avoid leaving baby to cry for more than ten minutes at a time – give him the reassurance of a brief glimpse of you.
- Pick baby up in the morning and after daytime naps as promptly as you can and while he is still happy; avoid using cot or bedroom as a punishment.

Sleep diaries

Some parents keep a sleep diary as a means of identifying, preventing or solving sleeping problems. If you are attempting to correct sleep disruption it can be particularly useful to record your baby's night-time behaviour and your own responses towards her, before planning any change.

10.30am	Put in cot for morning nap. Cried for a few minutes then fell asleep till 11.15.
2.00pm	Fell asleep for 15 minutes while in pushchair.
7.30pm	Fell asleep while breastfeeding. Put in cot.
10.00pm	Cried. Husband went upstairs to rock to sleep (unsuccessfully) eventually brought baby down for breastfeed. Wide awake then, wanted to play.
11.30pm	Put in cot. Cried so much we picked him up again.
Midnight	Fell asleep in arms. Put in cot.
3.00am	Woke for breastfeed. Fell asleep in our bed and was left there until
5.00am	Woke again, fed for two minutes. Fell asleep. Put back in cot.
7.30am	Woke and cried. Took dummy and fell asleep for another hour.

Extract from a sleep diary kept by the mother of Robert, an eight month old boy. The boy could already settle alone – for his morning nap – so the mother began to put him down awake after early-evening and late-evening breastfeeds. She decided not to take baby into bed as she knew he would fall asleep feeding. Two weeks after this was written, Robert was sleeping regularly from 9.00pm to 7.00am.

Time for change?

Many parents have found the ideas described in this handout work with just a little perseverance. If you think your baby's sleeping pattern should be changed, then choose a good time to start – not when you are especially tired or have visitors staying! Try to catch up on your own lost sleep by organising some alternative care for your baby for an hour or two on the first couple of days. Above all, do not struggle on alone – if you already have a sleeping problem in your family, whatever the age of the child, your health visitor should be able to provide the necessary advice and support, so that you too can enjoy some silent nights.

11

The hyperactive child: dietary management?

John W.T. Dickerson, PhD, FIBiol, FIFST, Hon FRSH, Hon MA PHA
Formerly Professor of Human Nutrition, School of Biological Sciences, University of Surrey, Guildford

The idea that behaviour disorders might be caused by food is not new. As long ago as 1945, Schneider suggested that 'allergy' played an important role in causing childhood hyperkinesis. Current interest in the possible role of diet in the aetiology of behavioural disorders stems largely from the suggestion by the late Dr B.F. Feingold that approximately 30 to 50 per cent of hyperactive children show a significant improvement in behaviour when placed on a special elimination programme (see Feingold, 1975). Feingold's work suggested that naturally occurring salicylates and artificial food additives may cause hyperkinesis in children with a genetically determined predisposition. Feingold's observations were extended to children with disruptive behaviour associated with learning disability, epilepsy and mental handicap. It is not surprising that these observations have caused concern to food manufacturers and paticularly parents of such children, who began to see in this industry and the complexity of food the cause of their children's problems.

What is hyperkinesis?
The terms hyperactivity, hyperkinesis and hyperkinetic syndrome are used loosely in both medical and lay literature. Clinical features include overactivity, inattentiveness, distractibility, poor tolerance of frustration, temper tantrums, impulsive behaviour, resistance to discipline, anxiety, aggression, cognitive dysfunction and learning problems. In some children the disorder is associated with epilepsy or some other neurological disorder and in America in particular children are often described as having 'minimal brain dysfunction'.

In the UK, the 'hyperkinetic syndrome' has been reported to occur in 0.1 per cent of children (Rutter et al, 1970), whereas in the US it is said to be present in four to 10 per cent of all school-age children. This difference is probably due to the criteria of diagnosis. From its very nature it is clear that psychosocial factors may be responsible for the condition. It is all too easy for parents and teachers to ignore this possibility and look for dietary or other factors to account for a child's unruly behaviour. Some of these children may be very intelligent and are simply frustrated.

Aetiology

Many factors have been suspected or presumed to play a role in the aetiology of hyperkinesis. Complications during pregnancy, smoking during pregnancy, genetic factors, environmental pollutants (particularly lead from car exhaust fumes), adverse reactions to foods, disturbances in the metabolism of the cerebral neurotransmitters dopamine and noradrenalin, as well as disturbances in parental-child interrelationships, have all been implicated. It is unfortunate, but not altogether unreasonable, that doctors faced with a child with this sort of problem may all too readily prescribe drugs, particularly amphetamine, methyl phenidate (Ritalin) and tricyclic antidepressants, with or without behaviour modifications, in attempting to treat the disorders. These treatments, particularly by the drugs, while ameliorating symptoms, do nothing to remove the cause of the hyperactivity. The possibility of undesirable side-effects cannot be ruled out.

Diagnosis

If a child is obviously hyperactive, attempting to identify the factors responsible may seem a forbidding, time-consuming task to which busy doctors feel unable to devote sufficient time. A nurse working in the community can make a substantial contribution in obtaining the necessary information for an accurate diagnosis. By visiting parents in their homes, and where appropriate, talking to teachers at school, she can help to obtain the necessary comprehensive appraisal of medical, social, educational and psychological factors (Varga, 1979). Typically, the child will have a history of abnormalities in the key temperamental traits mentioned above. It is important to determine how long the child has had symptoms. It has been suggested (Rutter et al, 1970) that 'hyperkinetic syndrome' be used only for children whose symptoms arise before the age of five years.

As infants (Weiss and Hechtman, 1979), hyperactive children may have been poor and irregular sleepers, and have had colic and feeding problems. Sometimes infants that develop hyperactivity have not enjoyed being held for more than a few minutes. Hyperactive toddlers are described as children who never walk but run, do not play with one object for more than a few seconds and who combine an impulsive behaviour with a lack of fear. When the child reaches three to four years parents complain that he is very demanding, does not listen and finds it difficult to play with other children. Parents despair that neither praise nor punishment is effective, that 'nothing works'. Not infrequently, parents will disagree as to what methods are most helpful.

It is not surprising that hyperactive children present considerable problems to teachers. Their behaviour will not only have a marked disruptive effect on class discipline but also lead to the underachieving of intellectual potential. If the child is naturally intellectually very 'bright', problems at school, as in the home, may be due largely to frustration.

It is only after all this information has been properly assessed attempts can be made to diagnose the cause of the child's behaviour problems.

Food and hyperactivity

The idea that food may be the cause of a child's difficult behaviour is attractive. It is something tangible that parents can understand and, theoretically, if the foods can be found and eliminated from the diet, the child should be better. The satisfactory testing of Feingold's hypothesis that a considerable amount of hyperactivity in children is caused by foods containing salicylates and additives, particularly colours, has proved difficult; reported studies are open to severe criticism with reference to the diagnosis and description of the children's condition, placebo control and dosage of additives (Rippere, 1983). It is difficult to accept that they provide a satisfactory basis for the confident statement by the US Nutrition Foundation that they "provide sufficient evidence to refute the claim that artificial flavourings and natural salicylates produce hyperactivity". There may be a real 'danger' inherent in the Feingold approach (Rippere, 1983) in that if omission of all food additives and salicylates is found not to result in improved behaviour it may be concluded that food is not the cause of the condition. The possibility must always be considered that any food may cause hyperactivity in a susceptible child.

There is a widespread belief that sugar (sucrose) causes behaviour and learning problems in children. These have been attributed to reactive hypoglycaemia or 'allergic' reaction. However, both these hypotheses remain at present untested and unproven (Ferguson et al, 1986). However, in relation to individual children, it may be prudent to retain an open mind on this matter because some children do like large amounts of sugar, which may be associated with hyperactive and aggressive behaviour in some.

Hyperactive Children's Support Group

The Hyperactive Children's Support Group (HACSG) has done much in the UK to help families with hyperactive children. It provides a list of foods suitable for hyperactive children which are salicylate- and additive-free. They also provide ideas for nutritious meals. A survey by questionnaire (Higgs, Colquhoun and Dickerson, unpublished) of 117 hyperactive children who had adopted the HACSG dietary programme showed that parents of over 90 per cent of the children claimed improvements in coordination, concentration, fits or tantrums and aggressiveness; over 50 per cent for crying or screaming; 82 per cent in speech; 73 per cent in disruptive behaviour; and 71 per cent in self-abuse. These results confirmed those of a previous study which had involved over 100 other children (Pepler, Colquhoun and Dickerson, unpublished). Taken together, these studies appear to offer support for the Feingold hypothesis. However, considerable caution is needed in their interpretation. First, they were obtained by questionnaire and it is very difficult to construct an unbiased questionnaire, particularly when parents are reporting on their children. Furthermore, the sample of parents who completed the questionnaire may well have been self-selected with mainly those parents who thought their children had benefited from the diet being willing to complete it. The new diet could have been a considerable nutritional improvement on the child's normal diet and the changes therefore have been due to improvements in general nutrition.

Furthermore, the possibility must be considered that putting the children on the diet resulted in an improvement in parent-child relationships, with the parents taking rather more interest in their children. However, bearing all these difficulties in interpretation in mind, it can be recommended with some confidence that parents of hyperactive children try the diet. It is nutritious, harmless, a good diet for all the family and might help to cure hyperactivity even though the precise reason for the improvement cannot be defined.

A more recent study (Egger et al, 1985) has confirmed that foods other than those suggested by Feingold can cause hyperactivity. In this study, 76 selected overactive children were treated with an oligoantigenic diet consisting of two meats (eg, lamb and chicken), two carbohydrate sources (eg, potatoes and rice), two fruits (eg, banana and apple), vegetable (eg, any brassica), water, calcium (calcium gluconate 3g/day) and vitamins (Abidec 0.6ml/day). The diet was adjusted to suit the taste and habits of the family, and to avoid any foods suspected of causing symptoms and those for which the child had a particular like or craving. A total of 42 children improved; of these, 21 recovered completely and achieved a normal range of behaviour. The results were confirmed in 28 other children by a double-blind, crossover, placebo-controlled trial in which foods thought to provoke symptoms were reintroduced. A total of 48 foods were incriminated. While artificial food colours and preservatives were the commonest provoking substances, no child was sensitive to these alone. The sensitivity of children to very specific foods is illustrated by the finding that sugar provoked a change in behaviour in nine of 55 children tested.

The nurse's role

Parents of hyperactive children need help, understanding and reassurance. A trusted community nurse or health visitor may be the best person to provide this, but she will work as part of a team. The extent of her role will depend on the child's doctor, the availability of dietetic advice and, of course, her own knowledge and interest. Doctors are not always sympathetic to parents who consult them about overactive children. In such cases it may be that a health visitor can pursue the matter herself by collecting the information on which a diagnosis can be based. In addition to their behaviour, information should be obtained about the child's usual diet and in particular any likes or cravings for specific foods.

All community nurses and health visitors should have sufficient knowledge to detect nutritional inadequacy in a child's diet, but if possible the matter should be discussed with a dietitian. If it is decided to proceed with an investigation of the child for reactions to specific foods, again this is best done with the help of a dietitian, with the nurse having an intermediary caring and supporting role. It is essential that testing is done as objectively as possible; a nurse in touch with the family in the home can be a great help in this. False positive reactions are often recorded. Careful testing can seem tedious but is essential if anxious parents are to be prevented from putting a child on an unnecessarily restricted diet in the hope of a 'cure'. It should not be forgotten that sometimes the cause of the problem is the parents' own behaviour towards the child.

References

Egger, J., Carter, C.M., Graham, P.J. *et al* (1985) Controlled trial of oligoantigenic treatment in the hyperkinetic syndrome. *Lancet*, **1**, 540–5.

Feingold, B.F. (1975) Hyperkinesis and learning disabilities linked to artificial food flavours and colours. *American Journal of Nutrition*, **75**, 797–803.

Ferguson, H.B., Stoddart, C. and Simen, J.G. (1986) Double blind challenge studies of behavioural and cognitive effects of sucrose-aspartame ingestion in normal children. *Nutritional Reviews*, **44**, 144–58.

Rippere, V. (1983) Food additives and hyperactive children. A critique of Conners. *British Journal of Clinical Psychology*, **22**, 19–32.

Rutter, M., Tizard, J. and Whitmore, K. (1970) *Education, Health and Behaviour*. Longman, London.

Schneider, W.F. (1945) Psychiatric evaluation of the hyperkinetic child. *Journal of Pediatrics*, **26**, 559–70.

Varga, J. (1979) The hyperactive child. *American Journal of Diseases of Childhood*, **133**, 413–8.

Weiss, G. and Hechtman, L. (1979) The hyperactive child syndrome. *Science*, **205**, 1348–53.

Useful addresses

Hyperactive Children, 150 Donvant Road, Killy, Swansea. Tel: 0792 201749.

Hyperactive Children's Support Group, 71 Whyke Lane, Chichester, West Sussex PO19 2LD. Tel: 0243 551313.

Handout: diet and hyperactive children

Foods suitable for hyperactive children

Any cereals without artificial colouring and flavouring.

All homemade bakery goods and sweets.

Bakery goods preferably made with 81–100% stoneground flours – plain or self-raising.

Shop-bought brown bread made from 81–100% stoneground flour.

All fresh meats, offal, poultry, and white fish.

Homemade ice cream, sweets, lollies, jellies made with permitted fruit juices.

Plain gelatin for jellies.

Bananas

Lemons

Grapefruit } Permitted as fruits and juices

Pears

Pineapple

Melon

Avocado pears

Homemade lemonade

Homemade or shop jam with permitted fruits but without artificial colouring and flavouring.

Pure honey.

Homemade puddings.

Plain yoghurt.

'7 up' drink.

Milk, eggs, white cheeses and unsalted butter.

Pure cooking oils and fats.

White vinegar.

All fresh vegetables.

Points to remember if your child is hyperactive

1. Overactivity is a complex condition. It can be caused by a number of factors, including environmental pollutants such as lead, and foods.

2. It is worth trying to identify the cause of your child's behaviour problem because if this is avoided your child could be much better.

3. You will need help if you are trying to investigate the problem. You should discuss the matters with your doctor and ask if it is possible to see a health visitor or dietitian.

4. In order to help your doctor, keep a record of your child's behaviour, and of his diet for three weeks.
   Especially note those things that are eaten frequently and those consumed between meals, such as ice lollies and coloured drinks.

5. Discuss the record with your doctor and/or health visitor.

6. You may be advised to submit your child to tests. The only tests that are worth considering are those that involve the elimination of certain foods from the diet. Other tests, such as skin tests or blood tests are unreliable.

7. Try to change to a diet based on wholefoods. The one suggested by the Hyperactive Children's Support Group is worth trying.

8. Keep in touch with your health visitor.

12

What are febrile convulsions?

Lorenzo C. Visentin, RGN, EMT
Staff Nurse, Paediatric Unit, New Cross Hospital, Wolverhampton

A child can produce a high temperature with a very minor illness, so it is not surprising that febrile convulsions occur in approximately 2.5 per cent of all children. Febrile or infantile convulsions are seizures that occur in the context of a febrile illness in a previously normal child (Brunner and Suddarth, 1986).

Febrile convulsions, as distinct from other seizure disorders (epilepsy, focal seizures and myoclonic fits), always accompany intercurrent infection such as pharyngitis, tonsilitis and otitis, and often simply coryza. The child presents with a core temperature of at least 38.8°C and an average age of 18 months, although these convulsions can occur at any time between six months and three years. It is rare to see febrile convulsions in a child over five.

As with all paediatric disorders, the convulsions cause the parents great anxiety. It is therefore essential that nurses offer and reinforce reassuring information to prevent undue anxiety, direct confrontation, in naturally concerned parents. Such anxiety can, in extreme cases, result in direct confrontation between parents and nurse.

Adverse events

Adverse events are harmful for children when they arouse more anxiety than the child can cope with. If a parent is anxious and tearful about the child being in hospital, this anxiety may be conveyed to the child and increase his or her distress (Davies, 1984). This makes parental education essential. The following handout is a simple, comprehensive guide to febrile convulsions intended for parents of children admitted to a paediatric unit. The information it includes gives the parents the opportunity to mentally rehearse a stressful event, so when it actually takes place there should be less emotional disturbance. A parent prepared for any care given to their child, either in or out of hospital, needs to feel in control of the situation. This feeling can be passed subconsciously through to the child, so the child then feels less distressed.

Parents of children admitted to hospital for febrile convulsions need help, understanding and reassurance – to them, their child is of paramount importance. As the convulsions occur only in the context of a febrile illness, the onset is likely to have been sudden with no predisposing factors other than a runny nose, so the parents are likely to be shocked by them. The first piece of reassurance anxious parents should receive is a warm welcome, while the child's safety is attended to.

Nursing action

Immediate nursing action involves reducing the child's temperature and preserving a patent airway. The child should not be restrained, and the convulsion's type should be accurately recorded, including its duration and severity. It is also important to give the parents an opportunity to become involved in their child's care. There must be a constructive discussion between the nurse and parents to establish what each expects of the other, where the gaps are and whose expertise fills them. If this is not done, it may be presumed that one or other is responsible for an aspect of the child's care and the gap is filled with frustration and dissatisfaction on both sides (Brewis, 1986).

It must be remembered that a common explanation for fever is misinterpretation of normal temperature reading (Brunner and Suddarth, 1986). Routine observation of temperature gives an ideal opportunity to teach parents the correct technique and how to analyse thermometer readings. Normal temperature ranges in children are:
- Oral   36.4 – 37.4°C
- Rectal   36.2 – 37.8°C
- Axillary   35.9 – 36.7°C

Parental guidance

Parents are likely to be the primary carers when the child is discharged home (Williams, 1987), so it is essential they are given a simple yet comprehensive guide to febrile convulsions; the recurrence rate is quite high – 40-50 per cent for a second convulsion and 15 per cent for a third. Verbal emphasis is needed as well as the written guide, especially when attempting to dispel old wives' tales such as sweating out a fever. Going through each stage of the guide with the parents gives them the opportunity to assimilate all the information they are receiving and to ask appropriate questions. Although time-consuming, the verbal reiteration of the information contained in the guide may be vital – parents do not necessarily have good reading ability, and those with a poor reading ability should be taken into consideration (Williams, 1987).

Once the child's condition has stabilised, teaching the parents simple first aid procedures such as the recovery position is useful. This easily learnt technique may appear complicated at first, but it is simple and may be life-saving. It is important to emphasise the need for non-restraint, to ensure parents are aware that they may unintentionally harm their child if they attempt restraint during a convulsion. When demonstrating how to maintain a patent airway, it is also important to tell parents not to force anything between the child's teeth. (Children occasionally bite their tongues at the onset of a convulsion, but will not damage it any further once the fit has started).

Recurrence

The high recurrence rate of febrile convulsions is influenced by a number of factors. The child's age is important, as the risk of recurrence is greater in younger children. There appears to be a familial tendency to convulsions, and those with a positive family history are more susceptible to recurring convulsions. Thirty per cent of recurrences occur within the first six months after the first seizure, and all recurrences (about 40-50 per cent of all cases) occur within 30 months. Girls are more likely than boys to have a recurrent febrile convulsion. Interestingly the risk of developing non-febrile convulsions is low (approximately 3 per cent) – children at risk are those with persistently abnormal electroencephalograms, central nervous system infections, prolonged febrile seizures (ie, above 20-30 minutes) and those who experience multiple febrile convulsions during one 24 hour period. Children who have this increased risk should be assessed and further guidance offered. Information leaflets are a cheap aid which can provide useful guidance and advice when properly explained (Williams, 1987), but they should never replace the specialised advice offered by paediatric nurses on a one-to-one basis with parents.

References
Brewis, E. (19860 Parental prerogatives.*Nursing Times*, **82,** 51,34–35.
Brunner, L.S. and Suddarth, D.S. (1986 The Lippincott Manual of Paediatric Nursing. Harper and Row, London.
Davies, C. (1984) Mother's anxiety may increase child's distress. *Nursing Mirror,* **158,** 18,30–31.
Williams, J. (1987) Home nursing for parents. *Nursing Times*, **83,** 19,53–54.

Handout: if your child has suffered a febrile convulsion . . .

Your child has suffered a fit with a high temperature – a febrile convulsion. This is always caused by an infection like a cough or a cold, and there is a chance that another convulsion may occur (although this only happens in half of all cases), but if you follow a few simple rules another convulsion may be avoided. This handout will help you both to avoid your child having another convulsion and to know what to do if this should happen.

Do's
Do take your child's temperature – leave the thermometer under the armpit for a full minute. Normal temperature varies slightly according to such things as the time of day, but it should fall between 36.5 and 37.5°C. If temperature is higher:

Do stay with the child – remember he or she may feel poorly and need comfort – also watch those open windows – accidents can still happen.

Do give a paracetamol syrup (such as Calpol) from the chemist, following the instructions on the bottle for the dose.

Do give plenty of drinks – with a little sugar added, as your child will be losing a lot of fluid by sweating, which must be replaced.

Do phone the family doctor, who will be pleased to see your child and may arrange hospital admission if necessary.

Do phone the children's ward. We will be happy to help and there is always a trained specialist nurse on the ward available for advice.

Don'ts
Don't insist on your child staying in bed. Children with a temperature don't always feel poorly and the bedclothes don't help bring down their temperature.

Don't listen to old wive's tales such as sweating out a fever – this is positively dangerous.

Don't hesitate to bring your child to casualty or direct to the children's ward.

Don't sponge your child with cold water, this will stop the temperature falling.

If your child has another fit

Remember, if your child does have another fit, that children almost always come out of it themselves – even if they go blue for a short time. There are a few things you can do to ensure safety:

1. Clear the area around the child to prevent any accidents.

2. Turn the child onto his or her side, into the recovery position.

3. Do not put anything into the child's mouth. Once the fit has started children do not bite their tongues.

4. Stay with your child but do not attempt to restrain him or her.

5. Dial 999 and ask for an ambulance.

For the future

It is extremely unlikely that your child will have suffered any permanent damage, and it is also unlikely that there will be any recurrence. By the time he or she goes to school, the chance of another fit will have all but disappeared. Do learn more about First Aid from one of the voluntary organisations such as St John's Ambulance Brigade, the British Red Cross or St Andrew's Ambulance Association (Scotland). Their number will be in the phone book.

Finally remember **if you are ever** **in any doubt,** **always ask and find out!**

Useful phone numbers Doctor... Children's Ward .... Health visitor..................................

13

Encopresis: family support must accompany treatment

Arthur F. Turner, BA, RGN, DNCert, Prof Prac Cert (Wales)
Service Centre Manager, University Hospital of Wales

For most parents the training of their child's bowels occurs between one and 2½ years of age. This is often initiated either due to family tradition or following advice from the family health visitor. By the age of four, 89 per cent of children will be totally in control (Largo and Stutyle, 1977). Despite this, constipation remains very common, and in certain circumstances encopresis can follow.

Much can be done to help encopretic children and their families by the primary health care team (or continence advisor). An individual care plan can be developed that supports the family as a unit, as many encopretic conditions can be exacerbated by ignorance and anxiety.

Influences prior to encopresis

Training for faecal continence is usually based on the gastrocolic reflex – the peristaltic wave that occurs after a meal that pushes faeces from the colon into the rectum, initiating the desire to defaecate. Many parents believe that sitting their young babies on a potty and thereby utilising these reflexes can potty train them. However, most children do not have the physical or mental maturity to be able to fully control their bowels until about 18 months old, so the potty training is for convenience only – although most people would agree that it is much better than cleaning a number of soiled nappies daily. Coupled to the potty training is an element of praise and encouragement which reinforces the child's approved behaviour (in this case passing its faeces in the potty) while the child becomes aware of the sensation associated with a full rectum.

There are many factors affecting the consistency of stools, and these can strongly influence the child's ability to become faecally continent. They include diet, amount drunk and exercise. If the stools are hard and consequently difficult to pass, the child may begin to associate the potty or toilet with pain and thereby learn a pattern of behaviour that contributes towards constipation and delayed learning of faecal continence. This delayed pattern of behaviour can also occur when there is a transition from the potty to the toilet. The child may feel much safer opening his or her bowels in the semi-squat position produced by sitting on the potty. The praise that normally went with the use of the potty is often abruptly halted, while the child is expected to open his or her bowels while teetering on an uncomfortable toilet.

The position adopted as a result is not ideal for the natural response of the body to close the epiglottis and lower the diaphragm in order to help the expelling of the faeces and assist the peristaltic contractions (valsalva's response). Children cannot produce much push if their feet are unsupported, so they need, as a basic requirement, a child's toilet seat, as well as somewhere to rest their legs.

Parental response

There is also a link between encopresis and the parents' response to soiled nappies when the child is very young. If the child only receives attention when he has soiled nappies and is otherwise unstimulated and neglected, this can give rise, when the child is older, to a pattern of soiling, psychologically learnt from babyhood to gain attention from adults. Although a strict toilet training regime at too early an age is not recommended, if the child is not introduced to the potty or toilet in a relaxed fashion soon enough, he can become used to passing faeces in a nappy, often preferring to become constipated than use the receptacle his parents have belatedly offered. This can begin to create the stress in toiletting activities that is so common in the families of encopretic children.

Another important facet to faecal continence is the availability of the toilet. Many household routines do not allow time for opening of the bowels, especially in the rush of the morning and this 'refusing the call to stool' is often responsible for defective excretory patterns later on in childhood. The rectum of such children becomes stretched and desensitised and this leads to a chronic condition of the bowel, where the bowel becomes grossly distended by the backlog of faecal matter. This blockage prevents the normal cycle of elimination and a spurious diarrhoea presents as liquid faecal matter and leaks its way around the obstruction. Diet has a strong influence on the normal workings of the bowels, as food high in roughage assists in the passage of the forming stool and makes defaecation considerably easier. Although some families have been giving their children too much dietary fibre, children in the main are allowed to be too conservative in their selection of food. The appeal of fast, convenient foods lures them towards a diet high in fat and lacking in fibre. Meals like beefburgers and chips are so popular with children that it is not surprising constipation is a common problem, and the setting up of constipation clinics in some health authorities highlights this (Bennett, 1988).

Encopresis

Encopresis, or faecal incontinence, is not a very common complaint but it gives rise to much more repulsion and distress than enuresis. One study suggested that it affected about one per cent of five-year-olds (Bellman, 1966), but a later study put the figure as high as 1½ per cent of seven to eight year-olds (Schaefer, 1979). This is only a tenth of the incidence of enuresis. Many of the studies that have been conducted into encopresis have highlighted the role of stress in the appearance and continuation of faecal soiling and many of the effective treatments concentrate on ways of removing anxiety from the child's environment. Much of this work has been done in England and will be described later.

Investigators (eg, Hussain, 1984) have tried to categorise types of encopresis, and while these distinctions are not mutually exclusive they do appear to give some framework to the professional to enable a rational form of treatment to be carefully thought out and implemented. The three types of encopresis are roughly:

1. The child who has never been trained who may come from a deprived family whose lifestyle mitigates against formal training.
2. The child may regress from continence after a period of faecal continence.
3. The child who has faecal incontinence/soiling due to retention and constipation.

Reducing stress

By far the easiest way of reducing stress (and the cornerstone of most of the treatment options that have been described involves the reduction of stress) is to try to get the parents or carers to praise the behaviour that they wish for from the child and to remove from their interaction with the child any form of retribution associated with the soiling or faecal incontinence. Implementing this however, is fraught with problems. It may be perfectly natural to get aggressive and short-tempered with a child that soils but it is the primary way of reinforcing his/her negative behaviour; in contrast, praise is one of the most effective forms of discipline. A programme must be formulated in order for a logical approach to treatment to be written down and the staff and carers involved must have a good idea as to the direction of that treatment.

Encopresis is often secondary to chronic constipation and very often these cases are extremely resistant to treatment. Some of the problems may be caused by the ignorance of the parents or carers as to the exact function of the bowel. This requires the practitioner to have a good relationship with the family so that a 'demystification' process can be undertaken (Landman and Rappaport, 1985). This is vital, and considerable time needs to be spent on it so the blame for the faecal incontinence can be shifted from the child to faulty toiletting habits. The shame of the parents can also be alleviated by highlighting the biological reason for their child's problem. Effective treatment can only be achieved by education – fear or distaste of faeces often initiates the disastrous chain of events so difficult to reverse.

Treatments

Relief of constipation   Hospital admission is best sought so that the deconstipation exercise can be achieved, although the constipation clinic that Bennett (1988) has described has a high community involvement in the treatment. The contact between the practitioner and the patient must be maintained even during the hospital phase of the treatment. The deconstipation routine can be achieved by the use of phosphate enemas; micro-enemas; mineral oil or ducolax.

It is less important, however, to persevere with one of the above agents as long as the regime is successful. Once the bowel is clear (and this can be checked by comparing X-rays of 'before and after') the functioning of the bowel is maintained by tapering the medication over a few months and a toilet routine which allowes for twice daily sittings!

With this sort of approach it is useful to allow the patient some scope for decision making as this helps his self-esteem and increases the chances of compliance. Studies have shown (Levine and Bakow, 1976) that there are certain children who would be likely to have the least success in this type of therapy. If the client records the following in their history it is doubtful if the treatment will be successful:

A.   Little stool retention at first.
B.   Soiling at different times of the day.
C.   Misbehaviour at school.
D.   A blasé attitude about soiled underwear.

These children should be considered for early recall and referral to other specialists.

Habit training   A second way of treating constipation-associated encopresis is to instigate a programme of habit training (Lowry, 1985). This involves the parents in much of the initial care. The bowel is cleared by the parents instilling a nightly enema. After this has been achieved the child should attempt to defeacate for 10 minutes after one or more meals. If the child fails at the end of the second day's attempts then an enema is again given, (eg, phosphate enemas).

This programme requires the parents to praise the child for successful bowel actions and accident free episodes while appearing fairly non-commital and calm about any incontinent episodes. The results achieved by such a programme are fairly impressive; over 50 per cent of the children become totally continent long-term with the number of incontinent episodes falling from 13.2 per week to 0.8 per week. Yet most encopretic children come from families where the stress level is extremely high and in such circumstances it may have been better to use a combination of recognised therapies such as structural family therapy and behaviour modification (Rydzinski and Kaplan, 1985).

By looking at the family as a cause of the child's disquiet and working on the areas of marital dispute and home-life disharmony that are causing the child's stress, great strides can be made in the treatment of this disturbing condition. Sharing the therapeutic tasks between husband and wife can often help to re-establish more balanced parental partnership towards the children. The couple together then can agree to be constant in their praise of the child when the desired behaviour is reached. This might be cold comfort to single parent families but it is often possible to involve other close friends of the family, or an older sibling might be prepared to help with the course of treatment.

Behaviour modification (Table 1) This can eliminate retentive encopresis very rapidly and has advantages over other methods of reducing the amount of parental involvement except for the integral praise for the desired behaviour. Despite the success of some of the

---

Behaviour modification   Three techniques can be used:

Gifts

The simplest of these is the giving of small gifts for unsoiled pants. This, however, has drawbacks in that it can encourage the child to become constipated to gain the desired gifts.

Overcorrection

This places a greater responsibility on the child, but still involves the giving of a gift. When the child soils he is required to wash out the soiled pants and 'practice' approaching the toilet from various directions and practice sitting on the toilet for a few seconds.

Negative reinforcement

By far the most successful technique experimentally, despite its apparent harshness:

1. After waking up, the child should sit on the toilet for 20 minutes or until a bowel action (whichever comes first).
2. Parental checks should be made every five minutes to ensure that the child is not allowed to do anything else on the toilet so he realises the purpose of the procedure. An effort can be made however to keep the child comfortable, for instance by supplying a stool on which to rest dangling feet. A bowel motion needs to be more, in bulk, than half a cup.
3. If no bowel action has occurred then the child has to stay on the toilet for 40 minutes after lunch or until a bowel action.
4. This procedure is then repeated following the evening meal for 90 minutes or until there is a bowel action. If the child has a bowel action, the daily pattern can be left for the rest of the day (Rolider van Houten, 1985).

Table 1. Behaviour modification.

above mentioned procedures, encopresis often requires a more detailed and integrated management philosophy so that the many strands of an individual's problem can be unravelled in a united professional way. An example of this unified approach has been developed by a team of doctors, social workers and physiotherapists from Aylesbury in Buckinghamshire (Wakefield, Woodbridge, Croke, Steward, 1984). Vital parts of this therapy are placed in the hands of the physiotherapists, teachers and play therapists to counteract the sort of natural peer revulsion and consequently damaged body-image of these encopretic children. An initial interview with the parents and child should be as informal as possible and although some practitioners like to see all the family together it may be an advantage to have the initial interview with the parents alone. It is often difficult to talk with a child present, and the value of a calm, reassuring first interview can be lost in the company of a distracting child. If the problem of the encopretic child is centred on a family-induced stress then this is often revealed at the first interview.

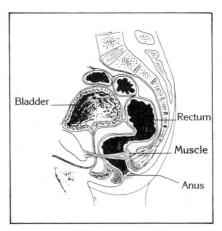

Figure 1. Position of bowel compared to other pelvic organs in the male.

Regime 1

Regime for the treatment of faecal incontinence –

Initial interview:
1st – Parents.
2nd – Parents and child.

Toiletting regime:
Visits to the toilet after meals and before bed and improved diet.

Physiotherapy:
Abdominal massage.
Yoga exercises.
Hydrotherapy – helps the child to regain his or her confidence in public.
Play-therapy – useful when working with the under 5s.

Medication:
Success is regarded as:
   No soiling.
   Bowel actions.
   Regular.
   No laxatives.
   Maintained for 12 months.

It is important to relieve as much anxiety as possible; diagrams (Figure 1) may help the child to understand the normal mechanisms of eliminating faeces. The child's often blasé attitude is explained as the most natural defence a child can employ given the seemingly unsolvable condition by which he is afflicted. An optimistic therapeutic climate must be maintained so that the most effective treatment can be pursued.

A toiletting regime should be instigated with the help of the parents. A star chart helps to keep a track of the child's progress, but it is not considered important in its own right. Despite that, some children do become continent during this period. Physiotherapists can reteach defaecation techniques by allowing the child to rediscover the normal workings of his body. High fibre food is emphasised as being beneficial against the damaging effects of fast food (Regime 1).

The benefit of getting the child to be aware of his body is highlighted by the emphasis on massage, yoga and swimming. These previously forbidden activities (due to the fear of soiling in public) being now allowed, greatly assist the child in reducing anxiety while enhancing confidence and a state of wellbeing. Yoga exercises are designed to help muscle tone of the bowel (to prevent constipation) and to help the child relax. Each exercise sequence should be carried out daily at home (Park Hospital, 1986). The sequence should begin with a 'tummy rub' for five minutes.

Intimacy

This intimacy between child and parent often makes vast differences in the quality of their relationship and usually the stress that was a barrier to the improvement of the encopresis disappears. Several points need to be emphasised. First, teachers and other non-medical professionals may be ignorant about the reasons for faecal soiling. This may lead to

---

Regime 2

Regime for management of retentive encopresis
1. Remove constipation by enemas, suppositories and laxatives.
2. Introduce a high-fibre diet.
3. Re-establish toiletting regime.
4. Reduce anxiety and increase parental support for the child.

Regime for management of non-retentive encopresis
A. Encourage talk about the problem.
B. Restore confidence in the child.
C. Allow the child to decide when to go to the toilet.
D. Reward for staying clean.
   i Love and affection and extra time for games when in a non-soiled state works better than:
   ii Sweets and rewards.

(Schmitt, 1984)

situations where children are banned from school swimming lessons, even though no soiling has ever taken place in the pool and it may be just because the teacher in charge of the swimming lessons has been made aware of the child's condition. The therapist dealing with the case should endeavour to explain the condition to the relevant people. Much of this work could be undertaken by a nurse with access to the help of other professionals. However, encopresis is a multifaceted condition which needs the cooperation of a number of professional groups linked in a fairly formal way. Thankfully nearly all retentive encopresis disappears by the age of 16 years, while only one per cent of nonretentive encopresis has an organic background. This remaining 99 per cent also resolves itself by the age of adolescence.

The programme for retentive and nonretentive encopresis have been identified by Schmitt (1984) (Regime 2). As has been detailed above there are many therapeutic avenues open to the therapist to help solve encopresis. Pressure to create opportunities to extend help to these children and their families must be applied in areas without any facilities for the care of these children and their families.

References

Bellman, M. (1966) Studies of encopresis. *Acta Pediatr Scan.*, **170**, 1, supplement.

Bennett, M. (1988) The fibre squad. *Nursing Times*, **84**, 4, 49.

Hussian, S.a. (1984) Childhood psychiatric disorders with physical manifestations. *Indian J. Pediat*, **51**, 205–216.

Landman, G.B. and Rappaport, L. (1985) Pediatric management of severe treatment resistant encopresis. *Dev and Behav. Pediatrics*, **6**, 6, 349–51.

Largo, R.H. and Stutzle, W. (1977) Longitutional study of bowel and bladder control by day and at night in the first six years of life, I: epidemiology and interrelations between bowel and bladder control. *Developmental Child Neurology*, **19**, 598–606.

Levine, M.D. and Badkow, H. (1976) Children with encopresis: a study of treatment outcomes. *Pediatrics*, **58**, 845–852.

Lowry, S.P. *et al* (1985) Habit training as a treatment of encopresis secondary to chronic constipation. *Journal of Paediatric Gastroenterology and Nutrition*, **4**, 397–401.

Rolder, A. and van Houten, R. (1985) Treatment of constipation-caused encopresis by a negative reinforcement procedure. *Journal of Behav. and Exp. Psychiat*, **16**, 1, 67–70.

Rydzinski, J.W. and Kaplans, L. (1985) A wolf in sheep's clothing? Simultaneous use of structural family therapy and behaviour modification in a case of encopresis and enuresis. *Human Sciences Press*, 71–81.

Schaefer, C.E. (1979) Childhood encopresis and enuresis: causes and theory. Van Nostrand Reinhold, New York.

Schmitt, B.D. (1984) Encopresis. *Primary Care*, **11**, 3, 497–511.

The Park Hospital for Children, Oxford (1986) Details of current therapy ideas and instructions to parents.

Wakefield, M.A. *et al* (1984) A treatment programme for faecal incontinence. *Developmental Medicine and Child Neurology*, **26**, 613–616.

Bibliography

Hill, P. (1991) Assessing faecal soiling in children. *Nursing Times*, April 3, **87** (14).

Jones, C. (1985) Encopresis. *American Journal of Nursing*, **85**, 154–156.
    A nursing article highlighting the fear-pain cycle.

Leoning Baucka, V.A. and Cruikshank, B.M. (1986) Abnormal defecation dynamics in chronically constipated children with encopresis. *The Journal of Paediatrics*, **108**, 4.
    A study highlighting the dangers of long-term constipation.

O'Regan *et al* (1986) Constipation – a commonly unrecognised cause of enuresis. *AJDC*, **140**, 261–1.
An interesting article linking enuresis with constipation.
Perkins, M. *et al* (1985) Diagnosis and management of constipation and encopresis in childhood. *Texas Medicine*, **81**.
A clear guide to enable an accurate diagnosis and sensible management programme.

Useful address
'ERIC' Enuresis Resource and Information Centre, 65 St Michael's Hill, Bristol BS2 8DZ. Tel: 0272 264920.

Handout: preventing constipation and faecal incontinence in children

Most children without physical and mental developmental difficulties will achieve continence of faeces by the age of four years. However, a few children do find it difficult, and most can be helped at home. This handout will help you prevent your child having problems in achieving continence.

Babies
Babies are extremely sensitive to your reactions from a very early age, so it is a good idea not to show abhorrence towards a soiled nappy, however unpleasant it is to clean up.

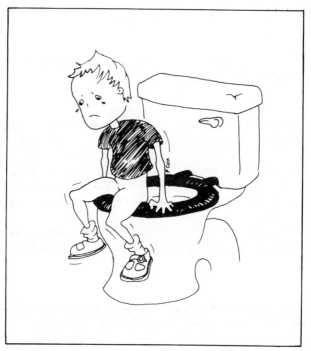

Children cannot produce much push if their feet are unsupported

Words
The words you use to describe anything to do with faeces are also important. They should not carry any sort of negative implication. For example: 'Number two' is better than 'Poo', and 'Poo' is better than

'Dirty'.

Any family words for faeces are acceptable as long as they are not used in a negative sense for other things.

The potty

From about six months on (or when your child can sit up comfortably without help) it is useful to introduce the potty after feeding. This provides a comfortable seat to hold the child in the best position to catch the gut movement that happens after each meal. If your child learns to associate the potty with a pleasant, enjoyable time, it will be easier to achieve continence (musical potties that play a tune when used can help!).

One year old

After a year (seldom earlier) children may seem more conscious of their bowels, either by showing displeasure at a soiled nappy or by asking to sit on the potty. It is often worthwhile letting them go without nappies at certain times of the day (when convenient) with the potty near at hand, so they can practise skills of holding on.

Praise

Always make sure you praise your child when he or she is successful, but make sure you do not criticise any accidents.

Toilet

After potty training, the next stage is toilet training. It is a good idea to have an 'open door' toilet, so your child can see (and can therefore mimic) older children and adults using the toilet. A small toilet seat to fit over the bowl, and a stool to rest feet on will make the transition from potty to toilet much easier (though some children like the challenge of holding themselves on the toilet). Bottom wiping and hand washing can be taught at this stage.

Children who have become continent for some time can become incontinent again as a side effect of either stress and anxiety or constipation.

Stress

It is impossible to completely avoid stress and anxiety in childhood, but major episodes such as starting school, moving home or parental disharmony can result in loss of control. This is best prevented by preparing your child well in advance for any predictable changes in his or her life. Nothing can compensate for a warm, caring relationship with parents to minimise stress.

Constipation

This can usually be avoided by making sure your child eats plenty of fibre, drinks plenty of liquid and has time to defaecate without being rushed.

Faecal incontinence (encopresis) affects one or two children in every hundred, and can usually be completely resolved by the age of 16, but carries with it feelings of great revulsion. Careful handling while your child is developing continence can avoid problems later, as can efforts to avoid constipation.

If your child does have problems, your GP will be able to refer you to an expert in this condition. This might be another GP, a district nurse, health visitor, continence advisor or pediatrician. They will be able to set up a programme to help you and your child to solve the problem together.

14

Childhood continence problems

Arthur F. Turner, BA, RGN, DN Cert, Cert Prof Prac (Wales)
Service Centre Manager, University Hospital of Wales

Childhood continence

Childhood continence can be acquired as simply as walking. Children learn through their accidents. Many people do not fully appreciate the complex sequence of events that precede full continence. The child needs to be able to register three vital aspects of his or her internal and external environment, namely:

- when he/she wants to eliminate;
- where he/she is expected to put it;
- how to get to the identified recepticle.

While most children become both urinary and faecally continent without any apparent effort, some children and their often distraught families suffer the anxiety of delayed continence skills (Woodmansey, 1967).

Urinary and faecal incontinence beyond the age where it is to be expected causes a great deal of stress within a family, and this often exacerbates the incontinence. Away from the specialist centre, the advice and practical help can be at best patchy and at worse non-existent. Before dealing with the problems, I will discuss the types of behaviour adopted by parents to influence the gaining of continence.

Toilet/potty training

Most parents/carers incorporate some form of training within their care, and the use of a potty is favoured by many, yet there are several ways in which parents feel that they can influence continence.

Laissez-faire   This technique adopts the positive view that most children reach continence without interference, and that the child itself will instigate the 'drying-out' process. However, problems can ensue because children sometimes will not pass their faeces into anything other than their nappy; preferring to be constipated rather than use a potty or a toilet to open their bowels.

Early potty use   Some parents, often influenced by the advice of their parents, use a potty to take account of the gastro-colic reflex and presume that the bladder works in the same way. Although some assume that the use of the potty illustrates a trained bladder, this is rarely so until about 18 months (sometimes earlier, often later) as physical and mental maturity is rarely sufficient before then (Cartoon 1). However, many parents/carers find it is beneficial for the child to develop an awareness of the potty as the place where urine and faeces are passed into, however slight this awareness may initially be. Anyone who has had umpteen soiled nappies to wash on a wet winter's day will understand that just one less can be a huge relief!

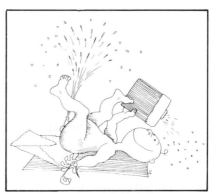

Cartoon 1. Children are rarely mature enough to train their bladder before 18 months.

Familiar play object   Often if the potty is introduced too late, the child will play with it and find it difficult to use properly, especially if it is introduced as a plaything, as some advise (Cartoon 2).

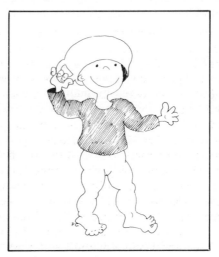

Cartoon 2. The child may find using the potty difficult if introduced as a plaything.

Rapid training Many parents find a rapid training method which consists of intensive potty education over either 24 or 48 hours very successful, especially when the child seems ready, for example, pulling at the nappy or asking to use the toilet like its parents. This may be appropriate at any age (18 months to three years) as long as the child is prepared to cooperate (Cartoon 3).

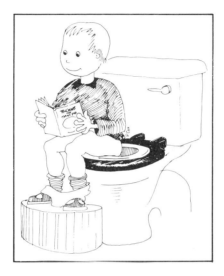

Cartoon 3. Rapid training may be appropriate if the child is prepared to cooperate.

Punishment and retribution Potty training can cause much aggravation especially when the parents are anxious to rid themselves of the chore of washing or disposing of nappies. The resultant stress often causes more or prolonged incontinence. The key to continence is a calm even-handed attitude linked with praise for the dry successes, rather than retribution for the failures. Learning is a process of adjusting behaviour by mistakes, and praise is a powerful form of discipline.

It must be stressed that the average age for achieving dry days and nights is three years (the figures vary slightly) and *only half* the children are dry at this age (Meadow, 1980). Continence development can cause family problems, however, as early as 18 months, especially if the parents/carers are anxious about the training regimen and feel a subconscious necessity to 'race' with families whose children of a similar age are continent. If the incontinence continues, help is best given after the age of four (Essen and Peckham, 1976) and more complex treatment is usually reserved for children who are over eight years old (Harvey and Kovar, 1985).

Stress and anxiety

Many incontinence problems are caused, made worse or even precipitated by stress and anxiety. This is just as true when the delayed development occurs at the age of 20 months as it is when the compounded stress emanates from a child's peer pressure at school. They can also be caused by the child having a psychological block about elimination (Robbins, 1985); many parents use the epithet 'dirty' to represent faeces, and our toilet habits are often shrouded in mystery and the British 'closed-closet' mentality, which can make children feel that they alone have this 'dirty problem'.

Types of incontinence

Nocturnal enuresis   This is common in three year olds but gradually the incidence deminishes with age until only 0.05 per cent of girls and one per cent of boys are still bedwetters at the age of 17 years (Figure 1).

There are now many techniques available which help to reduce the time taken for nocturnal bedwetting to resolve itself (Table 1).

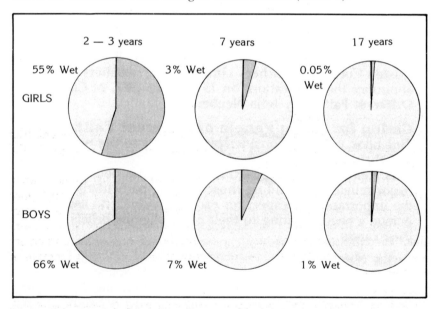

Figure 1. Incidences of nocturnal enuresis decrease with age (Sillitoe and Reed, 1986).

Diurnal enuresis   This occurs less frequently but is a particular problem among handicapped children. It is however, more intrusive and comes to the child's peers' attention much more easily and quickly.

The handicapped child   Handicapped children are especially vulnerable to a delay in learning. Continence often appears to be the least of the carers' problems initially but the discovery that the incontinence will continue beyond the 'normal' age of attainment is often a source of worry to the parents. Many problems, such as the poor provision of pads and the non-availability of a suitably educated professional can exacerbate an already difficult situation.

Encopresis and the management of bowels Faecal soiling again is amenable to a series of practical management techniques, but will also respond to alternative management such as yoga and massage. Much of the encopresis is thought to be due to stress, and alternative approaches such as yoga and relaxation, centre on the family stress (Landman and Rappaport, 1985).

Increased practitioner interest. Pad and alarm. Overlearning. Intermittent reinforcement (Pad and alarm). Dry Bed Method (Azrin, Foxx & Sneed). Hypnosis. Family Counselling (Clinical Psychology). Medication (Meadow, 1988).

Table 1. Treatments available for nocturnal enuresis.

Professionals and care

There are many professionals associated with the care of these children and sometimes the care can overlap or, more often, leave gaps, to the detriment of the child's treatment.

Continence attainment in childhood is fairly easily gained in most cases. However, it is also a source of stress within the family, and poor management in the first two years can lead to problems of a greater significance in the later years of childhood and adolescence. An even-handed, calm and relaxed attitude on the behalf of parents and carers can only assist children in both their normal and delayed attainment of continence.

References

Essen, J. and Peckham, C. (1976) Nocturnal enuresis in childhood. *Development, Medical and Child Neurology.* **18**, 5, 577–589.

Harvey, D. and Kovar, I. (1985) *Child Health – A Textbook for the D.C.H.* Churchill Livingstone, Edinburgh.

Landman, G.B. and Rappaport, L. (1985) Paediatric management of severe treatment resistant encopresis. *Development and Behavioural Paediatrics,* **6**, 6.

Meadow, R. (1980) *Help for Bedwetting.* Churchill Livingstone, Edinburgh.

Meadow, S.R. (1988) *Desmopressin in Nocturnal Enuresis.* Horus Medical Publications, England.

Morgan, R. (1981) *Childhood Incontinence.* Disabled Living Foundation: William Heinemann Medical Books Limited, London.

Robbins, B. (1985) The psychology of incontinence. *Journal of District Nursing.* 16.
Sillitoe, R. and Reed, S. (1986) Enuresis – dry at night. *Community Outlook,* March, 20.
Woodmansey, A.C. (1967). *British Journal of Medical Psychology,* **40,** 207.

Bibliography
Morgan, R. (1981) Childhood Incontinence. Disabled Living Foundation; Heinemann
   Medical Books Limited, London.
   A very practical book dealing with many problems that have been experienced by a
   knowledgeable and working therapist in childhood incontinence. Weak on references.

Useful address
'ERIC', Enuresis Resource and Information Centre, 65 St Michael's Hill, Bristol, BS2 8DZ.
   Tel: 0272 264920.

15

Bowel training for children with spina bifida

June Rogers, RGN, RSCN, DPNS, SN Cert
Special School Nurse, Springfield Special School, Kirkby, Merseyside

Spina bifida is a developmental defect of the spinal column in which the arches of the vertebrae fail to fuse. Present at birth, it is usually at the lower end of the spine but can occur anywhere from the back of the head to the base of the spine. There are two main types:

Spina bifida occulta   In this case, although there may be failure of one or more vertebral lamina to fuse at the midline, there is no cystic distention of the cord and meninges, and there is rarely any effect on function (Figure 1).

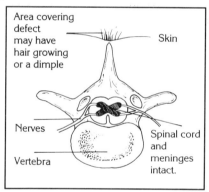

Figure 1. Spina bifida oculta.

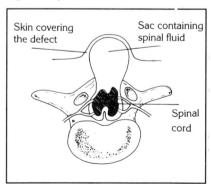

Figure 2. Spina bifida cystica (meningocele).

Spina bifida cystica   There are two types:

Meningocele The protruding sac contains only the covering membranes of the spinal cord and spinal fluid. The spinal cord is intact and the defect usually covered with skin (Figure 2).

Myelomeningocele This is the most severe type, as the spinal cord is involved, and may also be imperfectly formed. This results in severe neurological disability – paralysis of lower limbs and incontinence (Figure 3).

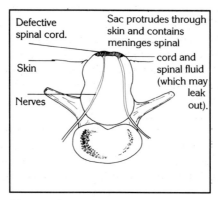

Figure 3. Spina bifida cystica (myelomeningocele).

If the spina bifida affects the segment of the spinal cord supplying nerves to the bladder, the child will be incontinent of urine. The damaged spinal cord will also be unable to pass messages up to and down from the higher centre in the brain concerned with voluntary control. The child is likely to have problems with bowel control as well, since nerves to the lower bowel and rectum will be affected.

With normal defaecation, the individual can suppress the urge to go if it is not convenient at that time – the defaecation reflex is able to be voluntarily inhibited. Children with spina bifida affecting their spinal cord are unable to control their bowels, resulting in faecal incontinence.

The Education Act of 1981 required local education authorities to review their educational provisions and identify the educational needs of children who may require special education. This meant that many children suffering from spina bifida could now be integrated into mainstream schools. However, this is a slow process, as many schools do not have the facilities to cater for handicapped pupils such as lifts and suitable toilet facilities. To this end and to increase the child's independence and social acceptance it was decided to evaluate the continence management of children with spina bifida, with emphasis on bowel control.

Bowel management

Over recent years the introduction of intermittent catheterisation has revolutionised bladder control and eliminated, in many cases, the need for indwelling catheters with all their associated problems. Bowel management, however, is often sadly neglected by the medical profession, and parents are left to muddle along by themselves.

It was decided to investigate bowel control in children with spina bifida and assess the different managements used, with the aim of evaluating the findings and developing a more structured management programme. Little seems to have been written on this subject, and what relevant papers were found were mostly from foreign journals.

With the aid of a grant from The Elizabeth Clark Charitable Trust, questionnaires were sent to 200 special schools, and various schools and centres were contacted and visited. Replies were received from 139 schools, only 70 of which had any children with spina bifida. This was due, in some cases, to the children having already been integrated into units attached to mainstream schools, while other schools catered only for children with a mental handicap. In all there were 581 children with spina bifida in the study. It was interesting to see the wide range of managements being used. Some schools appeared to put little emphasis on achieving bowel control, while others were obviously trying very hard to help the children achieve independence in this area.

Results of the questionnaire

Spina bifida can affect bowel control to varying degrees, so to get an overall picture of the problems the children were having, we wanted to find out how many were having problems with soiling and how reliable was their bowel control. The replies showed that just over half, 56 per cent (Figure 4a) of the children had little or no control over their bowels and 68 per cent (Figure 4b) had problems with soiling. Of the 581 children, 200 suffered from constipation and 48 had problems with diarrhoea. Despite the large number suffering from constipation only 64 were given a high fibre diet.

A wide range of medication was given to the children, mostly to relieve constipation. Lactulose was the most common – perhaps a change to a high fibre diet might be more beneficial. Only seven children were reported to be taking Loperamide, even though 48 had problems with diarrhoea. The following medications were also given – Bisacodyl, Celevac, Diocotyl-medo, Dorbanex, epsom salts, Laxoberol, Milpar, Senokot and syrup of figs.

Enemas or suppositories were given to 134 children on a regular basis and 114 had manual evacuations as a method of controlling their bowels, while 194 had no bowel management intervention whatsoever. Only 23 per cent of the children (Figure 4c) carried out their own management. Although physical and mental disability may prevent many of the children from becoming fully independent, I would suggest that, with training, the number of children able to participate in their own care could be increased. Only 42 per cent of the children had any active bowel management and only a further 12 per cent were encouraged to sit on the toilet at regular intervals.

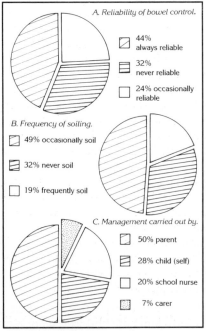

Figure 4. Statistics.

Neurogenic bowel problems

There appears to be two major problems with the dysfunctional or neurogenic bowel (Henderson and Synhurst, 1977): constipation and uncontrolled bowel action.

Constipation   In the normal process of bowel evacuation, the rectum fills and the nerve centres in the sacral part of the spinal cord facilitate a defaecation reflex, causing sigmoid peristalsis. Disruption of this process results in absent peristalsis causing rectal and colonic constipation, as well as uncontrolled passage of stool.

Chronic distention of the lower bowel can eventually lead to high faecal impaction, rectal prolapse, haemorrhoids, anal fissures caused by passing hard constipated stools, and perianal skin problems from chronic soiling. Management involves preventing the constipation and its resulting complications. Dietary management of constipation has the most benefit both to the child's health and in preventing constipation.

However, some children are picky eaters, and despite all efforts refuse to eat an adequate amount of fibre to prevent constipation. For these children and others where dietary management has failed, a more aggressive management is indicated, such as the use of laxatives and suppositories or micro-enemas.

Uncontrolled bowel action   This appears to result from deficiencies in the innervention of the striated muscles forming the external sphincter (Vigliario, 1980). Studies have shown that many of the children have normal reaction of the internal sphincter but absence of reaction of the external sphincter. Incontinence seems to occur when the pressure inside the rectum produces a reflex relaxation of the internal sphincter without sufficient voluntary control and reflex contraction of the external sphincter. On examination, the anus appears to be relaxed and the children have problems with repeated soiling.

If the conus medullaris is intact, however, some external sphincter action many be present. This can be tested for by pricking the skin around the anus with a pin, if the sphincter contracts, the nerves are intact. Even if the child has some degree of sensation, a number of other factors may interfere with him developing full control:

- Callipers or wheelchair may stop the child reaching the toilet as quickly as an able bodied child.
- Uncoordinated hand function will make the child slow and clumsy at unfastening his clothes and cleaning himself afterwards.
- Behaviourial problems such as hyperactivity will make it difficult for the child to sit on the toilet long enough to empty the bowel completely.
- Low ability may prevent the child from remembering a toilet training programme, without constant prompting and reminding.

Bowel training and management

Bowel management involves regular stool evacuations and scheduled toileting. This can be achieved by various methods, depending on the child. While some authorities advocate avoiding constipation at all costs, others induce constipation (Norton, 1986) by administering a constipating agent, and then induce a controlled evacuation by the use of an enema. It is important that each child is assessed, and the management programme adjusted to suit that particular child.

Although the methods by which the bowels are managed may differ, most authorities agree that scheduled toileting increases the chance of regulating the bowels (Vigliario, 1980). This involves sitting the child on the toilet at regular intervals at set times each day. The best time is after meals, especially breakfast, as it makes use of the gastric-colic reflex. The sitting position increases the intra-abdominal pressure and the child can be taught to improve this by grunting or trying to blow up a balloon.

Suitable toilet facilities should be available, ideally with enough room to enable the child to be able to transfer from wheelchair to toilet if necessary. There should be grab rails and supports so the child can sit safely on the toilet without the danger of falling off. A trainer seat is useful for smaller children, as is a moveable foot support. By trial and error, the following programmes proved the most successful:

The child who appears to have some degree of rectal sensation.

Avoid constipation, preferably by diet, otherwise use laxatives as necessary, always using the lowest effective dose. Encourage regular toileting, preferably after meals.

The child with sensation but external sphincter contracts to stimuli.

Avoid constipation as before and carry out controlled bowel evacuations using a micro-enema, the timing and frequency of which depends on the child. Alternate days seemed to work the best in this study, though some children need daily enemas to prevent soiling.

Some authorities also suggest giving a laxative, which stimulates colonic peristalsis, at bedtime. This usually acts in about 12 hours, in time to take advantage of the gastric-colic reflex after breakfast, when the enema can be given. However this regime may have to be adjusted to fit family schedules, especially if the mornings are particularly hectic.

The child with no sensation or reaction of the external sphincter.

In this case the anus usually appears lax and patulous. Management involves carefully induced constipation by administering Imodium (loperamide hydrochloride 2mg) or similar preparation, always using the lowest effective dose. A controlled evacuation is then carried out two or three times a week, either using micro-enemas or manual evacuations. However, since the advent of smaller disposable enemas, manual evacuation is becoming less popular, especially with the children.

The above management programmes are for use as a guide only, and will need to be tailored to each individual child's needs. Using these management programmes, we have achieved a very good success rate. However I have found any improvement, however small, is greeted with delight by both parents and children. In all cases prior to commencing a management programme it is important to ensure the child's bowel is clear – a straight abdominal X-ray may be helpful if there is any doubt. The following points should also be considered:

• Before starting encourage the child or parents to record stool frequency and consistency as this may be helpful in the management.

• Discuss and give a choice of management, if possible, with the child and parents. Decisions that are made freely are the most easy to accept and carry out over a prolonged period.

• Check the parents are fully aware of what is involved. Are they prepared to do or supervise the bowel management? Have they the time, or are they willing to give training every day if necessary?

• Each child must be treated as an individual and the chosen method must fit into the family routine.

• Background information is essential, try to be aware of the social conditions and related pressures. It may be necessary to involve other

agencies to provide suitable toilet facilities such as rails and raised seats.
• Liaise with other staff involved with the child. This enables both the child and parents to be given all round continual help and support, rather than conflicting instructions.
• If the child is admitted to hospital, ensure the staff are fully aware of the management programme to maintain continuity.

Improved control

The results of the questionnaire and research showed that there was greater incidence of bowel control achieved where some form of bowel management programme was carried out. The range of management carried out in the schools ranged from manual evacuations when a child continually soiled, with no other toileting, to almost full independence and bowel control in a college which used a programme of regular toileting and the administering of suppositories and enemas. However, the success of any bowel management programme hinges on the motivation of the child and parents. It is up to us, the professional carers, to provide that motivation.

References
Henderson, M.L. and Synhurst, D.M. (1977) Bladder and bowel management in the child with myelomeningocele. *Paediatric Nursing*, **3**, 5, 24–31.
Norton, C. (1986) *Nursing for Continence*, Beaconsfield Publishers, Beaconsfield.
Vigliarolo, d. (1980) Managing bowel incontinence in children with meningomyelocele. *American Journal of Nursing*, **80**, 105–07.

Bibliography
Bonnes, D.L. (1985) Spina bifida research study. *Curationis*, **8**, 2, 36–43.
   A comprehensive guide to issues relating to children with spina bifida.
Hodgkinson, K. (1982) Myelomeningocele – the spina bifida effect part 1., historical background. *Australian Nurses' Journal*, **11**, 9, 39–41.
Hodgkinson, K. (1982) Myelomeningocele – the spina bifida effect part 2, referral and assessment. *Australian Nurses' Journal*, **11**, 10, 31–33.
Hodgkinson, K. (1982) Myelomeningocele – the spina bifida effect part 3., discharge home on the first occasion. *Australian Nurses' Journal*, **11**, 49–52.
   These three pieces explain the background to spina bifida.
Pratt, L. (1984) Integrating the child with spina bifida into school. *Health Visitor*, **57**, 8, 242, 43.
   Mentions the role of the school nurse.

Acknowledgement
I would like to thank the following for their help and support. Joyce Wiseman, Mersey Region Research Nurse; Pat Webster, Alder Hey Children's Hospital; Sybil Deegan, Paediatric Continence Advisor, Newcastle H.A.; Pauline Young, West Berkshire H.A.; ASBAH. The children and parents who took part in my study, and all the school nurses who answered my questionnaire.

   Finally, my grateful thanks to all those involved in the Elizabeth Clark Charitable Trust without whose generous help and support I would not have been able to complete this study.

16

Let parents give the care: IV therapy at home in cystic fibrosis

Judith M. Ellis, SRN, RSCN, BSc (Hons)
Senior Sister, Medical Unit, Booth Hall Children's Hospital, Manchester

Booth Hall Children's Hospital runs a cystic fibrosis (CF) clinic for 140 children, 70 per cent of whom require a two week hospital admission every three months, to receive a course of intravenous (IV) ceftazidime. This entails a regular upheaval to the child's routine, which is entirely preventable if the parents are trained to administer the course of treatment at home. Since September 1986 parents have been receiving training on the ward, and 30 children now receive treatment at home.

Children with CF commonly have *Staph. aureus* in their lungs for which they permanently receive flucloxacillin orally, in an effort to limit lung tissue damage. Of the children treated at Booth Hall, 74 per cent also have colonisation with *Pseudomonas aeruginosa*. Once present, *Pseudomonas* is impossible to eradicate, and often undergoes a change whereby the organism itself produces highly viscid mucous, exacerbating the respiratory problems. *Pseudomonas* is not controlled by oral antibiotics, patients who are colonised receive IV ceftazidime (150 mg per Kg in 24 hours) for 14 days every three months to limit lung damage. This involves the siting of a cannula and administering the drug by infusion, over a 20 minute period at eight hourly intervals. Between doses the cannula and T extension set are heparinised with one millilitre of Hepsal. Four per cent of cases receive alternative antibiotic treatment because of ceftazidime resistance (Dinwiddie, 1986; Littlewood, 1986; David, 1984).

Why consider home therapy?
Hospital admission is a frightening experience for any child and it has been suggested that if prolonged or regular, it may cause long-term psychological damage (Bowlby, 1971), as well as creating other related problems for the child. For example, with patients' ever increasing life expectancy, an objective of care should be to avoid interference to their schooling.

The National Association for the Welfare of Children in Hospital's (NAWCH) Charter clearly states that "Children shall be admitted to hospital only if the care they require cannot be equally well provided at home." Children with CF face enough hospital visits and admissions without admission for treatment that could be given at home (Table 1).

Cause	% of all admissions	Average duration of stay (days)
Major respiratory infections requiring intravenous antibiotics.	37%	16
Other medical (liver disease, failure to thrive, diabetes, cor pulmonale, pneumo-thorax, meconium ileus equivalent).	20%	7
Minor respiratory infection (not requiring intravenous antibiotics).	12%	5
ENT surgery (polypectomy, sinus washout).	12%	4
Investigations of symptoms, confirmation of diagnosis.	9%	3
Social reasons.	5%	5
Coincidental conditions (epilepsy; asthma).	5%	4

Table 1. Causes of admission to hospital in children with CF (Booth Hall Hospital, 1979–81).

Every hospital admission is not only an upheaval to the child's life but to the whole family. Many parents want to stay with the child, making employment impossible, while daily visiting can be restrictive and extremely exhausting. The life of siblings is also disrupted so it is not only the child with CF's development and behaviour that is affected.

Parental rights to give all possible care to their child is now accepted in many paediatric centres (Brewis, 1986; Wootten, 1987). A system of primary nursing aids this approach, as it allows a holistic assessment of the child, family and the social context in which care is delivered.

Nursing intervention now also puts less emphasis on purely instrumental care. Orem (1959) identifies an educative, developmental approach, helping the parents to meet the therapeutic care demands – administering IV drugs to their child. Careful selection of suitably motivated and capable parents is vital. However, the parents' right to be offered training remains and precedents do exist – parents of children with haemophilia administer IV Factor VIII, and in America parents of children with CF administer IV drugs at home (Wery et al, 1984).

Instrumental care is not necessarily better implemented by admission to hospital:

- Ceftazidime is most beneficial if given at regular three monthly intervals. At home there would be no reason for any delay to coincide, for example, with school holidays or bed availability.
- To keep the circulating drug concentration at a constant therapeutic level requires regular eight hourly administration, which is easier to accomplish at home than on a ward, where staff shortages often mean doses are given hours late.
- Physiotherapy should ideally be given as soon as the child wakes up and just before bedtime – in hospital, it is given mid-morning and mid-afternoon, and so can be less effective.
- The hospital environment itself can be hazardous for the child. Children commonly pick up respiratory infections, especially pathogens such as respiratory syncytial virus or adenovirus.
- Admitting a child to hospital for two weeks is expensive.

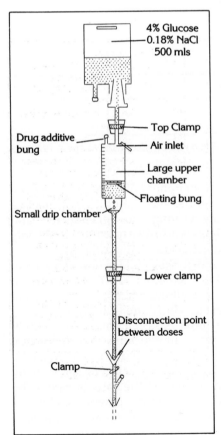

Figure 1. Equipment used – a diagram for parents.

How the system was implemented

A meeting was arranged with staff from other paediatric and adult CF units as well as with a leading paediatric haematologist. The feasibility of such a scheme was agreed and after further discussion at Booth Hall, certain essential criteria were identified (David, 1986).

1. It would be necessary to obtain the permission of every child's GP before training commenced and as part of his or her consent, the GP must agree to prescribe the ceftazidime.

2. The cannulas would be sited, and if necessary resited, in a hospital paediatric unit.

3. For the foreseeable future, all practical advice about home treatment and support would be given by the hospital staff.

4. Only medical staff and experienced nursing staff with the appropriate extended role working on the CF ward would train parents.

5. Written, specific guidelines would be compiled, stating clearly the correct procedure, hazards and dangers of IV therapy so that the parents were known to fully understand what they are doing.

Preparation of the Giving Set		
Step No	Hazard No	
1		Wash hands.
2	8	Check bag of fluid – clear, in date and sealed.
3		Remove outer wrapping.
4		Open giving set box – leave set in.
5		Close the 2 clamps, one to Chamber other on the line.
6	6	Remove top needle cover – DO NOT TOUCH.
7		Remove blue tag from bag.
8		Push needle into opening, touching neither.
9		Hang bag up.
10		Turn air inlet to open.
11		Open top clamp and allow 30 mls fluid into chamber.
12		Close top clamp.
13		Gently squeeze small lower chamber until 1/3 full.
14		Open bottom IV line clamp and watch fluid run through line. Continue until all air bubbles have gone. Close clamp.
15	6	Do not remove cover from end IV line until needed.

Table 2. Excerpt from procedure for giving IV antibiotics.

10. IV refuses to run:

(a) Check site – ? inflamed, swollen, excessively painful, then STOP, and ring for advice.
(b) Check clamp on extension set is off.
(c) Check air inlet tap above chamber is open.
(d) Check "bung" in chamber is floating. If not gently squeeze small chamber.
(e) Check IV bag high enough.
(f) Turn IV ling clamp off. Bend tubing below clamp level. Straighten and restart.
(g) Straighten arm or wrist, stroke cannula site.

11. Blood running down tube:

(a) Check air inlet tap above chamber open.
(b) Check bung in chamber is up. If not gently squeeze small chamber.
(c) Check IV bag high enough.

Table 3. Excerpt from procedure to recognise and act upon hazards.

Parental support

Parents are supported in caring for their child by a number of documents used to back up the help given by nursing staff.

The procedure   The first document explains the complete procedure stage by stage and is accompanied by a diagram (Figure 1). This ensures staff teach the parents in an identical manner. Hazard numbers are listed by each stage (Table 2) so if parents encounter a problem, they can refer to the list (Table 3).

The guidelines   These clearly set out the use of ceftazidime in CF including dosage, suitability and correct eight hourly administration. They also inform parents of the rigorous restrictions on acceptability for original training, as well as reminding them that at any time the hospital – or they themselves – can revert to hospital treatment. This will occur if their technique when observed giving the first dose of a course of ceftazidime is poor, if the child's condition warrants admission or if for family reasons they request admission. All possible dangers of IV therapy are outlined with guidance on how they can be avoided, recognised and acted upon as well as when to seek medical assistance.

Training record   When parents commence training, a record is kept of their progress, stating areas of difficulty and expertise as well as a running total of doses administered by each parent. The parents are continuously observed and at the end of each admission, summaries of their progress and future training needs are compiled.

Record card   This provides instructions for parents administering ceftazidime at home, and ensures the child's condition is monitored throughout the two week course, to aid decisions about future treatment. At clinic the child is weighed and the dose calculated, then instructions for reconstitution and administration are written on the card.

   To monitor the child's progress, the parents are asked to keep a record of the severity of his or her cough, amount and colour of the sputum and the best of three peak flow recordings morning and evening. The child's expected peak flow is written on the card at clinic. There is an additional space for comments on the child's condition as well as any problems encountered with the treatment. These record cards are returned by post. During the two week course, two sputum samples are sent for microscopy, culture and sensitivity.

Choosing suitable families

To be accepted onto the training programme, the family must meet certain criteria. Their suitability is not discussed until they have expressed an interest. Other criteria are:
- There are no active psychiatric problems in the family.

- The family must have their GP's consent.
- The family must live within easy travelling distance of a centre able to resite cannulas.
- They must have a clear understanding of the importance of all CF treatment, and particularly ceftazidime therapy.
- The family arrangements must make it feasible to give treatment at eight hourly intervals.
- There must be involvement of two care givers, so that the whole scheme is not reliant on one person.
   The child's suitability depends on a number of factors:
- The child's health must not require inpatient observation.
- The CF must be stable enough not to require other hospital-based services such as physiotherapy or dietetic advice.
- Staff must believe that the child will cooperate with and have sufficient trust in his or her parents.
- The child must have a patent cannula *in situ*.

Training families

Once the family has been chosen, their GP receives a letter asking for approval and when a reply has been received, training commences. Two admissions are usually required to reach the necessary standard but parents vary widely in their abilities. Eventually most parents trained so far have become confident and proficient in performing the procedure to the degree that it is believed that minor interferences in concentration (such as a phone call or the doorbell ringing) will not interfere with their performance. With the large number of children on the ward receiving IV ceftazidime treatment, these training admissions also provide an opportunity for the parents to learn what to do if the procedure does not run smoothly.

   Once it is felt that the parents are performing the procedure safely and confidently, they can be expected to respond correctly to any problems and they have a good understanding of basic principles, they are discharged home. The family then visit clinic every six weeks, and when a course of ceftazidime is decided upon, the record card is completed in clinic, the family are sent to the ward to have the cannula sited and for the parents to be observed administering the first dose.

Problems

As previously stated, before any training for home administration of IV ceftazidime can be considered, the approval of GPs must be obtained. Most agree immediately but some are apprehensive, giving reluctant permission, or in a few cases refusing. This is understandable, as with any form of treatment until it has been well established.

   Training the parents is extremely time consuming, especially in the early stages where it can take one-and-a-half hours to prepare and administer one dose, and on the ward only certain members of nursing staff have the necessary extended role. This means that occasionally due to lack of available time or staff with the correct extended role, parents have had to miss a session, which can cause friction.

A further problem is that junior medical staff called upon to administer ceftazidime are unwilling, due to lack of time and experience, to observe the parents. The teaching role has therefore fallen exclusively onto the nursing staff. This training programme has been important in standardising and improving techniques generally on the ward so that there is continuity in training methods.

Siting cannulas has also become a problem as only 8 per cent of the children treated at Booth Hall live within the district, with several residing outside the region, making it impossible for them to return to Booth Hall too frequently or quickly enough. If parents from other districts are considered, contact has to be made with their local general paediatric unit. One family discovered their GP's husband was an anaethetist and willing to help, and another adolescent patient's family learnt to insert butterfly needles to administer each dose.

At the commencement of the scheme there were unfortunately no community nursing staff specifically linked to Booth Hall CF Clinic. In 1988, a drug company agreed to finance the establishment of a CF Community Sister's post. This appointment has had a definite effect (Cleary, 1988; Whiting 1987). Selection for training has been streamlined, with a home visit to assess the parents and discuss the guidelines, prior to acceptance onto the scheme. The availability of support means single parents are now also eligible for consideration, the length of training has been shortened and terminally ill children, who may benefit from a further course of treatment can be offered this without it necessitating a hospital admission at a time when the family is so interdependent. However, with such a wide geographical area to cover this appointment cannot provide universal availability.

Obtaining equipment is a problem, with a disappointing response from approaches to the pharmacist and district nursing services. This has meant that currently, all equipment apart from drugs is provided from the ward, costing £84 for a two week course. Since ward budgeting is practised at Booth Hall, this expenditure is currently under discussion. It must be remembered however, that although this cost seems enormous, compared to the cost of two weeks' inpatient treatment, it is nominal.

Tactfully declining home treatment in families who want it but are felt to be unsuitable can be difficult, and this task has been undertaken only by the senior ward sister and consultant. So far, however, no family has reacted badly to this news and in some cases it seemed to be a relief, as they appeared to know their own limitations or unsuitability. The parents are never made to feel they have been wrong to ask, and they understand that they should feel free to ask again.

Many parents have never broached the subject, and again are not made to feel that it is expected of them as good parents. Other parents are seen to be suitable but their children are unable to cope at present with the strict regimen the parents must follow to administer IV drugs safely – for example, they may object violently if their cannula is touched. Some of these conflicts are due to the child's stage of development, and if this is the case the parents are allowed to carry on practising observed so that when staff feel the whole family is ready they will be proficient and can be discharged home.

With adolescent patients the problem is reversed. The children are more experienced, following many admissions, than their parents who have probably never been resident and are approaching it afresh. In this situation the children are excluded from the preparation stage until the parents are confident enough to cope with criticism.

The final problem throughout has been trying to decide who is responsible if anything untoward happens when the parents are administering the treatment at home. This probably accounts for the delay in starting such a scheme. "Reasonable care" must have been taken to avoid anything going wrong with home intravenous therapy. Reasonable care was defined by the Deputy Secretary of the Medical Protection Society as "what you and I think is reasonable, and what our colleagues consider reasonable". We feel the selection and training protocol provides this.

Limiting the effects of CF

By December 1989, 35 families were administering IV ceftazidime to their children at home. We feel that by training parents to be primary care givers, and only admitting children when it is absolutely necessary, we are limiting the adverse psychological effects of treatment on the child and its disruption on the whole family.

References
Bowlby, J. (1971) Attachment and Loss: Vol. 1. Penguin, Middlesex.
Brewis, E. (1986) Parental prerogatives. *Nursing Times*, **82**, 51, 34–35.
Cleary, J. (1988) The needs of children in the community. *Senior Nurse*, **8**, 6, 5–6.
David, T.J. (1984) Ceftazidime in Children with Cystic Fibrosis Ceftazidime a Clinical Perspective. Excerpta Medica, Amsterdam.
David, T.J. (Ed) (1986) Cystic Fibrosis in Children. Practical and Legal Aspects of Intravenous Antibiotics and Administration in the Home. Excerpta Medica, Amsterdam.
Dinwiddie, R. (1986) Management of the chest in cystic fibrosis. *Journal of the Royal Society of Medicine*, **79**, Suppl. 12, 6–9.
Wery, K. *et al* (1984) Home intravenous therapy: a management option for the patient with cystic fibrosis. In: Lawson, D. (Ed) Cystic Fibrosis Horizons. John Wiley & Sons, Chichester.
Whiting, M. (1987) Options in the care of acute childhood illness. *Nursing*, **3**, 23, 865–69.
Woolten, V.L. (1987) The care by parent unit. *Nursing*, **3**, 24, 897–99.

17

Understanding 'glue ear'

Vanessa Martin, SRN, RSCN
Ward Sister, The Queen Elizabeth Hospital, KIng's Lynn, Norfolk

The insertion of a grommet for 'glue ear' remains the most frequent operation performed on children under general anaesthetic (Donaldson, 1987) so it is not surprising that the majority of parents and primary school children have heard of 'glue ear' and of grommets. Many do not really understand the condition, nor the function of a grommet, however because it is difficult in a busy outpatient clinic to explain adequately why we treat a nose or throat infection, or a nasal allergy when the child has been referred with a hearing problem. Parents ask why ear drops are not offered, why operations are delayed or why they vary from child to child. Many parents become confused, and this can lead to misunderstandings and lack of cooperation.

Diagnosis

Glue ear is a condition in which sterile fluid accumulates in the middle ear. The main clinical feature is a conductive deafness which may go unrecognised by the parents but be picked up on routine audiometry, which has been performed in schools since the 1950s, or by recognition of the presence of fluid in the middle ear by a general practitioner. In spite of intensive research in the last 15-20 years, the aetiology remains uncertain. What is known is that there is "eustachian tube dysfunction and defective ventilation of the middle ear", and the pathology of the middle ear mucosa shows a "hyperplasia of the mucous glands" (Cowan and Kerr, 1986).

Glue ear is not a new condition (Black, 1985a). Clear descriptions are documented from as early as 1860s, and there is some evidence of earlier recognition. Black (1985b) reports that there were many suggested causes, ranging from infant bottle feeding, lack of physical activity and poor hygiene to poor bowel habits and violent nose blowing. Today the most common theories are viral infections, allergy, unresolved acute otitis media, and adenoidal hypertrophy causing obstruction to the eustachian tube and consequently to the drainage. Eustachian malfunction causes glue ear in 90 per cent of children with cleft palate, claim Cowan and Kerr (1986), though other otologists may have different theories. This means that the medical treatment for this condition can vary tremendously.

Surgery

Children who fail to respond to medical treatment are offered surgery, which may include removal of the adenoids, a myringotomy (making a small radial incision into the tympanic membrane) and removal of the 'glue' by suction, and/or the insertion of a grommet. While adenoidectomy is a controversial form of therapy for treating glue ear, insertion of a grommet is generally agreed to have benefits (Donaldson, 1987). Ideally, it is inserted for as long as the eustachian tube fails to function, as its aim is to temporarily replace it, but this period is difficult to predict.

Insertion of a grommet maintains hearing, ventilates the middle ear, leads to the recovery of the middle ear mucosa and, according to Stangerup and Tos (1986), has a positive effect on the process of pneumatisation. Their survey suggested that children with glue ear who are treated with grommets develop a significantly larger mastoid cell system. On the other hand, Black (1985a) states that "the use of tympanostomy tubes may possibly cause long term harm. In one study nearly half the children who had tubes inserted were found to have tympanosclerosis of the ear drum in the year or two after operation". Surgical treatment remains controversial.

As the above description illustrates, glue ear is a highly complex condition. The handout opposite is designed to outline the disease and possible treatments in a simple and concise form, free from complicated medical terms, although it cannot answer every question parents might ask. It can be photocopied and distributed freely to parents at the time that surgery is suggested.

Controversy

Even with the declared intention of simplicity, we can not avoid controversy. The care of a grommet is also debated by otologists. It seems to be widely accepted that swimming is allowed. The hole in the grommet is small enough to keep water out, and Smelt and Yeoh (1984) say that children with grommets inserted are no more likely to develop otorrhoea if they do swim than if they do not. Whether children's ears should be protected during hair washing is uncertain. Marks and Mills (1983) say that soaps and detergents, by lowering the surface tension, make water more likely to enter the middle ear. Protection of the ear for hair washing is included in the handout even though some otologists may feel this unnecessary.

References

Black, N. (1985a) Glue ear. The new dyslexia? *British Medical Journal*, **290**, 1963–65.
Black, N. (1985b) Causes of glue ear: An historical review of theories and evidence. *Journal of Laryngology and Otology*, **99**, 953–66.
Donaldson, J.D. (1987) Otitis media update *Journal of Otolaryngology*, **16**, 221–23.
Marks, N.J. and Mills, R.P. (1983) Swimming and grommets. *Journal of the Royal Society of Medicine*, **76**, 23–26.

Cowan, D.C. and Kerr, A.I.G., (1986) Paediatric otolaryngology. Secretory Otitis Media, 145–48.

Smelt, G.J.C. and Yeoh, L.H. (1984) Swimming and grommets. *Journal of Laryngology and Otology*, **98**, 243–45.

Stangerup, S.E. .and Tos M. (1986) Treatment of secretory otitis and pneumatisation. *Laryngoscopy*, **96**, 680–84.

Bibliography
Cotton, R.T. and Birman, C.W. Zaizal G.H. (1984) Serious otitis in children: medical and surgical aspects, diagnosis and management. *Clinical reviews in Allergy*, **2**, 329–43.

East, D.M. (1984) A layman's guide to grommets. *British Medical Journal*, **289**, 1596–98.

Shan, N. (1975) Glue ear – information for parents. Available from The Royal National Throat Nose and Ear Hospital, London.

Acknowledgements
I would like to thank B.P. Cvijetic, FRCS, and N.P. Chowdary DLO, for their help and advice, Norman Spooner for her practical and secretarial help, Ann Osborne for finding relevant articles, and Sarah Oldfield for typing this manuscript.

Handout: understanding 'glue ear'

In a normal ear, sound waves pass down the ear canal and through to the inner ear by vibrating the ear drum and ossicles, which are small bones in the middle ear. The inner ear then transmits those sound to the brain.

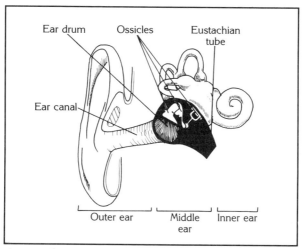

A normal ear

In glue ear, the sound waves can not pass through the middle ear because of a sticky glue-like fluid which prevents the ear drum and the ossicles from vibrating.

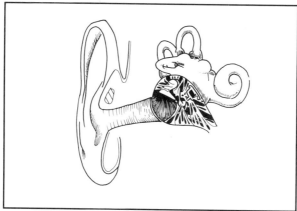

Glue ear

The purpose of a grommet

A grommet temporarily takes over the function of the eustachian tube. It allows air to enter the middle ear and gives the ear the opportunity to recover. Different grommets are selected to stay in place for different lengths of time. Some come out on their own after a few months, some remain for longer, and others have to be surgically removed.

If a short-term grommet has been inserted but the 'glue' collects again, it may be necessary to insert another type of grommet.

Why does this happen?

The eustachian tube, which runs from the middle ear to the back of the nose, opens on swallowing and allows air to enter the middle ear. Glue develops because the eustachian tube is not functioning properly.

Causes

The causes of poor function of the eustachian tube are not always clear. Repeated infections, enlarged adenoids, allergies or weakness of the muscles in the area of the eustachian tube can all contribute.

Treatment

The following may be tried:

- Antibiotics to clear infections.
- Decongestants to unblock nasal passages.
- Removal of adenoids, which lie at the back of the nose near the openings of the eustachian tubes.
- A myringotomy – making of a small hole in the ear drum and removal of the 'glue' by suction.
- The insertion of a grommet into the ear drum.

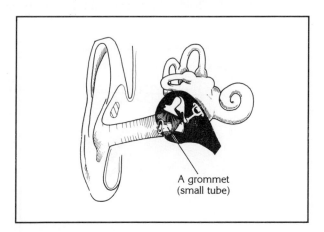

A grommet
(small tube)

Looking after a grommet

(1) When washing your child's hair, it is preferable if you place a piece

of cotton wool smeared with vaseline into your child's ear hole (entrance of the ear canal.) This is because soapy water can irritate the ear.

(2) Your child may swim, but do not allow him to swim under water, or dive.

(3) If your child should develop a discharge from his ear, or severe pain, contact your GP.

(4) You will be asked to attend the out patient department for a follow up. The surgeon will check whether the grommet is functioning and with the aid of a hearing test, will check that your child continues to hear normally.

Glue ear that is not treated

The condition of 'glue ear' is likely to improve in your child from the age of seven to eight years onwards. However, if persistent 'glue ear' is not treated before this time:

• The child may be slower to learn and to develop because he is not hearing properly.

• Changes may occur in the ear drum and the middle ear resulting in permanent deafness.

Useful contacts

Ward ....

Phone ....

Ward sister/Charge nurse ....

18

By accident or design: home accidents and young children

Eileen Thomas RGN, RHV, MA(Ed)
Special Projects Manager, Southampton Community Unit, Southampton

During the past ten years there has been a dramatic awakening to the major causes of death in children. Epidemiologists tell us that from six weeks of age to one year, most children who die will do so as a result of the Sudden Infant Death Syndrome (Jones, 1989). This tragic condition, which strikes usually without warning and when the infant is sleeping, has touched the consciousness of most parents of young children.

Once children have passed their first birthday the danger from this silent killer is thought to have passed. Except lying in wait is another cause of mortality which will claim more young lives than any other cause well into adulthood (OPCS, 1989). However, as one 1981 Lancet Editorial put it "to count deaths is not enough", because more children will attend hospital as a result of morbidity from this cause than those attending Paediatric Outpatients' Clinics (Golding, 1986).

Accidents have been termed "an endemic of epidemic proportions" (Silbert, 1975), with more than 700 children losing their lives each year in England and Wales (OPCS, 1988).

The loss of a young child is a tragic event which is thought to cause the worst form of grief reaction in the surviving family. In some parents their relationship is so damaged by their bereavement that they cannot remain as a couple, and separation and divorce are common in this group (Murray Parkes, 1983). Following research into Post Traumatic Stress Syndrome in children who survive or even witness a serious accident, significant and long-lasting emotional sequalae have been observed (Alexander, 1990).

Even when an injury is relatively minor, the tears of a frightened child may be matched by those of a frightened guardian. The words "if only", a doleful outward expression of the guilt a caring adult experiences, are frequently heard by Accident Department staff, Practice Nurses and Health Visitors, *after* the event. In terms of physical and psychological pain, accidents are almost immeasurable. The financial and social costs are, however, the subject of a national research programme by the Child Accident Prevention Trust.

Painful as it may be, to be wise after the event, the key to reducing this unacceptable toll of death and injury, lies uneasily with the knowledge we have gained *after* the incident has occurred. Study of the statistics relating to accidents in childhood has taught us the where, when, why, and what so necessary for prevention.

Where do children have accidents?
There is a well held belief that the home is the safest place to be. Well held but incorrectly so, more accidents occur at home, to all age groups, than in any other place (CAPT, 1989). People at the extremes of the age range are most at risk from home accidents, in part because their lives tend to be home-centred.

In 1976, the Department of Trade and Industry (DTI) started to maintain information on home accidents. The Home Accident Surveillance System (HASS) still collects data from 22 hospitals in England and Wales. It is from this source, together with research conducted by the Child Accident Prevention Trust (CAPT), and the Royal Society for the Prevention of Accidents (ROSPA), that most of our knowledge about home accidents in childhood has been obtained.

The vast majority of accidents to children under five years will occur in their home or garden (Alwash and McCarthy, 1987). After this age, the road represents the greatest danger to children under fifteen years, with pedestrian and cycling activities causing the most trauma (Constantinides, 1988). Within the home situation, the living room has been cited as the place where children are most vulnerable to injury (Alwash and McCarthy, 1987), but data from a Southampton study shows clear differences depending upon the type of accommodation occupied. That is, if a family have just one room as their main home, the bedsitting room will represent the most danger, with the most dangerous items such as kettles and irons concentrated in one very small area.

The families that are usually found in Houses of Multiple Occupation (HMIs) tend to be those with the lowest incomes and as such are at risk from a whole range of conditions (Constantinides, 1988). The Black Report (1980) showed clearly the relationship between poverty and ill health, a situation that has not changed with time. Since the poorest in a population tend to live in the most built up areas with the worst housing (Mitchell, 1984), these would be the locations to target accident prevention campaigns.

In Southampton, statistics relating to accidents in children under five years of age, have been analysed since 1983 (Thomas, 1989). These have clearly demonstrated that the areas where families are the poorest are also those where children are most vulnerable to accidental injury.

When do children have accidents?
Just as it is almost possible to predict the areas where the accidents will occur to children, enough is now known about the hour, day and month when they will be more probable than others.

During any normal day, the hours that produce the most attendances at Accident and Emergency Departments are those which are among the busiest in most households in England and Wales, namely mealtimes. Picture the parent, preparing food, managing one or more children of different ages, and in the wings – an accident just waiting to happen. Breakfast time and between 16.00 and 18.00 hours are those in which the most accidents occur to children in the home. Friday evening, the weekend begins but it also marks the start of an increased number of young casualties attending hospitals. School holidays, which are generally associated with relaxation are also the times when children will injure themselves more often (CAPT, 1989). Accident and Emergency staff refer to the 'Silly Summer Season', expecting large numbers of young victims to attend to during the months of July and August.

Why do children have accidents?

Children must live, according to one author, in "a world designed by adults for adults" (Bernfenstam and Kohler, 1981). The design of houses and their high technology contents do not adapt easily to little people with limited dexterity. The grown-up world is a truly perilous environment for a curious youngster, who simply must explore the strange big world in order to learn about it. Accidental injuries in childhood are phenomena which occur primarily in the industrialised nations (Pearn, 1978). It seems that as we make our homes more sophisticated we also make them much more hazardous for our children.

Everyday domestic items are not by law allowed to be dangerous. However, in the hands of an inquisitive child, almost anything can be potentially harmful. In a large proportion of childhood accidents, the event itself will be caused simply because of the child's normal development. That is, each new skill in order to be refined must first be practiced many times. The first step a child ever takes is the result of new balance and limb coordination.It is likely to result in a tumble and there is no child on earth that does not learn from getting up and starting all over again. Childhood accidents can be linked, especially in children under five years, to stages of developmental ability, which can teach us a great deal about the kind of accidents the young will sustain.

What kind of accidents do children have?

An examination of the accidents occurring to children shows a strong tendency to being age specific. Therefore some knowledge of the normal processes of child development is useful.

Under six months of age   All infants who are under six months of age are totally dependent upon the responsible adult for their safety. As a consequence, most of the accidents that occur to children within this age group will do so when the adult is nearby. A child will, with very little prior warning, reach out for a cup of hot tea, just as in the previous moment he or she had reached for a bright toy.

After an accident to a child under six months of age, parents will usually say "I didn't know he could do it", such is the dramatic speed of developmental progression. Under six months of age, the majority of accidents will be caused by falls and scalds (Colver *et al*, 1982). At six months of age, a proportion of children are beginning to move around, in particular boys who also have a higher rate of injuries than girls at all ages (Rivara *et al*, 1982). Such motor ability leads to the pulling-up stage and with it the risk of objects falling down onto the child. Scalds and burns remain an important cause of injury in this age group, but other kinds of accident such as falls from greater heights become significant, together with ingestions of virtually anything of a size that is possible to swallow.

The one year old child
The one year old child will have learned that even when hidden from view, objects remain permanent. They will remember and search for things such as bottles and, with enhanced manual dexterity, will often be able to open them. Grandma's handbag, so often the source of treats may also harbour her medication. Cough linctus, with its bright colour may seem just like a favourite drink and even the contents of full ashtrays may be worth a try.

The two year old child
Children of two years well earn the title of the 'terrible twos', since most of the adult world will seem just about within reach. They will try to imitate a great deal of adult or older sibling behaviour, but still do not have the strength or agility to undertake many activities safely. The garden and outside seem to be places of real excitement and the two year old, with his or her tantrums and tirelessness, can easily escape a weary parent's consciousness – for just that one moment.

Three years and beyond
From three years of age until fifteen, falls cause the most injuries to children, but they tend to become more severe with advancing years. The ten year old child is much more likely to break a bone following a fall since they tend to fall from greater heights, or from fast moving play objects such as skateboards and bicycles.

Road traffic accidents result in the greatest mortality in childhood, but in the home, burns and smoke inhalation cause the greatest loss of life (CSU, 1983). Even when it is not fatal, burns result in the most prolonged periods of hospitalisation for young children. A burn, as a function of the damage done to the skin, is never painless but one that may require years of distressing treatments to a growing child. Data from the Southampton study showed that, of all the children attending hospital as a result of scalds, 40% were because of spills from hot tea or coffee. In addition, 78% of attenders who were scalded were aged under two years (DPHAP, 1990).

Head injuries and lacerations result in the highest number of attendances at Accident and Emergency Departments in England and Wales. However, in the first instance, the term ranges from a severe injury involving a fracture to a bump, where the worst damage done is wounded pride. The vast majority of head injuries are minor with the child being detained in hospital as a precautionary measure. Cuts and lacerations tend to be more serious with increasing age when the child involves him or herself with more dangerous adult items such as tools.

In one London study, poisoning was the second most common cause of child casualty following falls. This research showed that some 46% of poisons were found in a handbag (Alwash and McCarthy, 1987). Another study of child poisoning victims found that, of the homes of 600, only 4% of medicines were kept in a locked cupboard (PAGB, 1987).

In England and Wales in 1988, 54 children died as a result of drowning and of these deaths, 65% were under five years of age (CAPT, 1990).

Actively preventing accidents to children

Our knowledge regarding the what, when, why and where of childhood accidents means that we are able to begin to actively prevent them. This anticipatory model will enable nurses and other professional staff to look for opportunities to support parents and guardians in the prevention of accidents to their children. It means being aware of age specific accidents and the time of day they are most likely to occur. One way of putting this message across would be by filling the space on the walls of Accident and Emergency Departments and Paediatric Outpatient Clinics with pictures linking accidents to a child's developmental ability.

Of all the conditions of childhood, the costs of accidents are among the highest, but so the opportunities for prevention are the most challenging.

References

Alexander, D.A. (1990) Psychological intervention for victims and helpers after disasters. *British Journal of General Practice*, **40**, 345–8.

Alwash, R. and McCarthy, M. (1987) How do child accidents happen? *Health Education Journal*, **63**, 235–57.

Bernfenstam, R. and Kohler, K. (1981) Proceedings of Methods and Experience in Planning for Accident Prevention.

Child Accident Prevention Trust (1989) *Basic Principles of Child Accident Prevention*, CAPT, London.

Child Accident Prevention Trust (1990) *Child Safety Review 3*, CAPT, London.

Colver, A.F., Hutchinson, P.J., and Judson, E.C. (1982) Promoting children's home safety. *British Medical Journal*, **285**, 1177–80.

Constantinides, P. (1988) Safe at home? Children's accidents and inequality. *Radical Medicine*, Spring, 31–3.

Consumer Safety Unit (1983) *Domestic Thermal Injuries: A Study of 1100 Accidents*. Department of Trade and Industry, London.

Department of Health and Social Security (1980) *Report of the Working party: The Black Report*. HMSO, London.

Director of Public Health Annual Report (1990) *Community Statistics*. Southampton and South West Hampshire Health Authority.

Golding, J. (1986) Accidents. In: Butler, N.R. and Golding J. (Eds). *From Birth to Five*. Pergamon Press, London.

Jones, D.A. (1989) Sudden infant death syndrome. *British Medical Journal*, **298**, 959.

Mitchell, J. (1984) *What Is To Be Done About Illness and Health?* Heinemann, London.

Murray Parkes, C. (1983) *Bereavement*. Penguin, Harmondsworth.

Office of Population and Censuses Surveys Mortality Statistics Series (1989) *Cause 1987 Series 14*. HMSO, London.

Office of Population Censuses and Surveys Occupational Mortality (1988) *Childhood supplement 1982–83 Series DS No 8*. HMSO, London.

Pearn, J. (1978) Predisposing factors leading to child trauma. *Journal Epidemiology and Community Health*, **32**, 190–3.

Predisposing factors leading to child trauma. *Journal Epidemiology and Community Health*, **32**, 190–3.

The Proprietary Association of Great Britain (1987) *Accidental Poisoning in Childhood: A Survey*. The Proprietary Association, London.

Rivara, F., Bergman, A., LoGerfo, J. and Weiss, N. (1982) Epidemiology of childhood injuries: sex differences in injury rates. *American Journal of Diseases in Childhood*, **136**, 502.

Silbert, J. (1975) Stress in families of children who have ingested poisons. *British Medical Journal*, **3**, 87–9.

Thomas, E. (1989) Accidents will happen. *Nursing Times*, **85**, 26–9.

19

Care of bereaved children: helping reduce psychosocial impairment

Ann Couldrick, RGN, FEATC, HV Cert
Bereavement Services Manager, Sir Michael Sobell House, Churchill Hospital, Oxford

Caring for a dying patient with cancer induces uncertainties in professional carers at all levels. Never more so than in caring for the dying young parent who is leaving needy children. This uncertainty can disable us so much that the very family that needs most support, can receive least from us, the professionals.

From supporting young families associated with a hospice over the last 10 years, and from listening to many staff themselves bereaved in childhood, the following strategies, which can be implemented before and after the death, will help to minimise psychosocial impairment and are worth considering.

Before the death

Include the children   Tell the children what is happening, that the sick parent has this illness called cancer and that everything is being done to make it go away. If death seems inevitable it is better to acknowledge that mummy or daddy is not getting better, but that everyone is trying very hard.

Minimise separation   Seeing is believing. Oncology wards with high radiation levels can present a very real problem and heighten the importance of getting Mum or Dad home. But wherever possible, allow the children to come as close as they want to. They know their own limitations, they may want to pop in and out of the sick room, and may seem heartless in their desire to escape but this is better than being kept away. Their fantasies about what is happening may be much more terrifying than the reality. The dying parent may want the opportunity to express their love and sadness. They may want to 'collect' some things that have been precious to them for the child to treasure. 'Mummy's box' that contains a favourite poem, a brooch, a photo, is a tangible link with the parent who has died. To mourn effectively, all human beings need to have a lost object. A parent who simply disappears leaves a child in a world coloured by unresolved mourning.

Encouraging a child to keep a scrapbook, to draw and to share their drawings, can help with understanding their inner world.

Direct parental attention   Sometimes the carer may be so taken up with all that has to be done, that they are blinded to the children's behaviour. Ask for each child, what might their understanding be of the situation? Is school going alright? Are they sleeping, eating, bed wetting, dreaming? Small children may claim this attention by 'acting out' their distress. For example, Lucy aged 5 started taking other children's things during the last three months of her father's life. The teacher handled it sensitively and helped the mother recognise that Lucy was feeling very helpless and shut out.

Mobilize resources   Are there are other members of the family who can be included? Are there any particular neighbours who could be asked to help if only they knew what was happening? Does the local church run a good neighbour scheme that can be alerted? Does the school know what the child is coping with, what the situation is at home? Could any help be obtained from Social Services (Family Aid, home help, playgroup, financial assistance)?

Reassure the children   Children need reassurance that they are not responsible, that cancer is not catching and that they are very important and will be cared for. Provide opportunities for the children to express their fears and feelings. "It must be very hard seeing mum so poorly," can often allow a child to realise that his or her needs are being recognised even if he or she does not respond directly. Convey to the child that he or she matters to you too, not just the person who is sick. Children who have lived through this experience have expressed bitterness about being ignored by the professionals who came in and out of their homes but ignored them.

Include them in the care   Children are great sources of comfort. There are many tasks that they can undertake if given the opportunity and access to the sick room: preparing drinks; massaging – children understand touch better than we do – they only need permission; reading to the sick person or being read to; snuggling up for a nap; and combing or brushing hair. All of these have been recollected by children whose parents have died, as being very precious things that they were able to do.

Help parents to be honest   We communicate with children whether we mean to or not. Our body language, our facial expressions, the tone of our voice often convey what we find difficult to verbalise. Leaving them to make sense of what is happening is cruel. Difficult things need to be rehearsed. How to tell a child that a beloved parent is dying may be facilitated by encouraging the parent to try it out on a steady, loving professional.

How much to tell and when, are difficult enough when the parent fully understands the prognosis so the parent will want to be as sure as possible that he or she knows what is happening. This is why it is so important for the staff to be consistent in what information they are giving.

It is also important to check that you have understood a child's question, following their lead is a good rule. As in sex education, a step at a time seems to be important, checking their understanding, for they will let us know when they have switched off and do not want to talk any more. Breaking bad news takes time and can often be eased by finding out what the child understands. "You must be worried by what is happening to Mummy" may elicit from the child what he is already thinking about. One father found that saying to his children aged 5 and 8 years old, "I'm worried that Mummy is not going to come home from hospital," produced the response quite naturally, "do you mean that Mummy is going to die?" Then they were able to talk about the uncertainty. He felt that by preparing them before the death helped them to accept other difficult things that had to be said later and that they trusted him.

Support the carer   If the person doing the caring can rely on support, knows how to get in touch, he or she will be much more confident in handling the children's uncertainties. This is almost certainly the greatest crisis of his or her life. To be isolated, unsure of support, uncertain when and from where to seek help, not only disables, but may make it impossible for the parent to respond to the needs of the children.

After the death
Whether to say goodbye to the body   This must be the decision of the parent, but if asked it seems important to say that many children who have lived through this experience, say that they were glad they were able to say goodbye or that they were sad that they were not given the opportunity. They do need preparation, a chance to choose, and explanation that the sick body that is left is no longer needed. Parkes says that the process of grieving for someone who has died, is to make real within us an event that has taken place outside us. Again, seeing is believing.

Attendance at the funeral   Again, many people looking back to childhood when a parent died, say how much they wish that they had been allowed to share in this family opportunity of saying goodbye. Understanding what happens at the funeral, why we bury or cremate the body, is important but may be very difficult for a parent to tackle. It seems to help to say that the body that we are putting in the ground or are burning, does not feel anything any longer. It is not feeling pain, cold, is not hungry or hurting. One 8 year old boy thoughtfully explained to his younger brother that he thought that "dying was like pricking a balloon, the air goes somewhere else, but we can throw the balloon away because you can never use it again." It seems to help to have a trusted adult there to give the children his or her full attention throughout the occasion, and this frees the mourning parent to experience it fully whilst at the same time, giving them all a common focus for their sadness.

Be available to discuss, explore questions   Children may have questions that they sense the parent who is left will not be able to answer. It can be very helpful to the parent to have professional support after the death. Many parents are relieved to feel that they are not going to be abandoned to the children's questions.

Older children may have very real fears that the drugs killed their mother or father, that not everything possible was done or even that the dead parent could have recovered if they had wanted to. Giving permission to explore upset, even angry feelings, can help the family mourn together.

If questions about the afterlife emerge, being sensitive to the family's religious beliefs but being honest about any uncertainty is not wrong. "Some people believe that we will be together again eventually" may be a fitting response but where there is no belief, it seems to be helpful to say that you do not know what happens or that "perhaps what is important in a person, are his talents, his kindness, his sense of fun, which seem to be passed on to you the children, so that nothing is lost." It does seem that children under 8 years have a clear belief in continued existence after death, whatever the family belief system.

It may be helpful to suggest to children before they go to sleep, that they close their eyes and with their 'inside eyes' picture Mummy or Daddy. Often they will tell you about the place they have visualised, a child 'saw' Dad sitting in a sunny field outside their tent. It was important for him to find a place to connect to in his thoughts.

Support the school   School teachers are with children for half their waking day and can be of enormous support. Making contact with the teacher and listening to their anxieties, can be very helpful to long-term care of the children. It is often after the death of a parent that the school's staff are very receptive to exploring their own uncertainties and they value contact and support.

Mobilise resources for the family   The primary health care team with its access to social services, community psychiatric services and volunteer groups will welcome having their attention drawn to the bereaved family. The local religious leader may already be involved, but if not he or she may be a stalwart addition to long-term support.

Reassurance   Children feel responsible in many ways for bad things that happen within the family. They may need it putting into words that this is not so. They did not make Mummy or Daddy ill or die, however naughty they thought they were, nor can they catch cancer themselves. It may have a cause, but mostly we do not know it, and they cannot have caught it. They will need reassurance that they will be cared for and that the parent who is left is unlikely to die too. This insecurity is natural and should be acknowledged. Many single parents have found it very helpful to explain to the child what other arrangements they have made in the event of their being ill or dying. It may seem cold blooded to put this into words, but many children straightforwardly ask these questions.

Within a week of his father's death, James, aged 10 years, the eldest of three boys asked his mother "What will happen to us should you have a car accident?" Fiona and Sally, six and four years old, found it difficult to let their mother go out in the evening until they were sure she had made arrangements for their future care. "You see, Mummy," said Fiona, matter of factly, "we don't feel safe any more."

Finally, having written information available that explores the understanding of children according to their age and development is very helpful to a parent. To this Couldrick (1990) has written a booklet *Grief and Bereavement: Understanding Children* for parents. It can be purchased from The Study Centre Coordinator, Sir Michael Sobell House, Churchill Hospital, Oxford.

My thanks go to my colleagues and the many volunteers who have worked with the bereaved over the years for sharing their experiences so generously. To the survivors of the tragedy of losing a parent in childhood, goes gratitude for teaching us how it really feels and for confirming the endurance of the human spirit in not only overcoming loss, but transcending it.

Bibliography
Black, D. (1978) Annotation of the bereaved child. *Journal of Child Psychology and Psychiatry*, **19,** 287–92.
Bowlby, J. (1980) *Attachment and Loss: Sadness & Depression*. Basic Books, New York.
Furman, E. (1974) *A Child's Parent Dies*. Yale University Press, London.
Glizer, E. and Kaffman, M. (1983) Factors influencing the severity of childhood bereavement reactions. *American Journal of Orthopsychiatry* **53,** 668–76.
Grollman, E. (1967) *Explaining Death to Children*. Beacon Press, Boston.
Hilgard, J., Newman, M. and Fisk, J. (1960) Strength of adult ego following childhood bereavement. *American Journal of Orthopsychiatry* **30,** 788–99.
Jewett, C. (1984) *Helping Children Cope with Separation and Loss*. B. T. Batsford Ltd, London.
Krementz, J. (1987) *How it Feels When a Parent Dies*. Victor Gollancz Ltd, London.
Masterton, J.F. (1976) *Psychotherapy of the Borderline Adult: A Developmental Approach*. Brunner Hazel, New York.
Osterweiss, M., Solomon, F. and Green, M. (1984) *Bereavement, Reactions, Consequences and Care*. National Academy Press, Washington DC.
Raphael, B. (1984) *The Anatomy of Bereavement*. Hutchinson, London.

20

Rooting for the source of anxiety: child psychotherapy at work

Dorothy Judd, BA, Dip. Art Ther., Cert. Ed., MACP
Principal Child Psychotherapist, Oncology Department, Middlesex Hospital, London and Visiting Teacher, Tavistock Clinic, London

Child psychotherapy aims to help children, even very young children, to rework unresolved emotional conflicts. All children experience conflict, anxiety, and trauma in response to their families and the world around them, as well as inner struggles over growing up and coping with aggression, frustration, separation and loss. This is often felt at an unconscious or fantasy level, and may be expressed through play.

Objectives of child psychotherapy

Child psychotherapists help children who have been subjected to adverse experiences or show emotional difficulties to share and explore aspects of their unconscious internal world. The child's mood, play, drawings, body-language and speech are carefully observed and experienced by the therapist, while any anxieties which may interfere with the child's development (often originating in early experiences) are directed towards the therapist, as are positive or loving feelings. This phenomenon, called transference, is one of the central forces in any therapeutic relationship with both children and adults. Indeed, the safe and sequestered nature of the setting, the regularity of the sessions, and the therapist's interpretations of the transference of feelings make it an intrinsic 'tool' of the treatment.

Clearly the 'vehicles' of communication children use are usually very different from those of adults, so the technique, equipment and setting for child psychotherapy also differ. However, child psychotherapists whose qualifications are recognised by the NHS work on psychoanalytic lines, and their theoretical framework is basically that of psychoanalytic psychotherapists working with adults. Child psychotherapists can be Kleinian, Freudian, or Jungian, or a combination of these 'schools', depending on their training, and will have to undergo personal psychoanalysis. In work with adults, it is generally the 'child within the adult' that is identified for treatment; with children, the young child or baby part of the self is often more accessible. Children can, however, be haughtily indignant when their 'baby feelings' or 'baby needs' are addressed, especially when they are consciously struggling to be more grown-up and to resist regressive pulls towards earlier infancy and dependence. These earlier phases of development, though, may not have been adequately worked through.

Children of course, unlike adults, do not volunteer for treatment, nor do they necessarily acknowledge the need. Adolescents generally need to be prepared to attend and to allow the process to begin, while younger children have less choice in this matter. Carers are usually responsible for initiating an assessment, bringing the child to the sessions and supporting the treatment, even in the face of resistance. However, children generally enjoy and value the experience of being really listened to and made sense of, and often do not want sessions to end.

Child psychotherapy in practice

One case study illustrates the benefits of child psychotherapy. In a psychotherapy session, Paul, aged 14, complained about his school bag being full of holes. He had come for weekly psychotherapy since his disclosure to the child psychotherapist five months previously that his mother and older brothers had been beating him. This was investigated and validated by social services, and Paul was taken into care. He had originally been brought to child guidance by his mother, at the suggestion of their GP, for his persistent stealing at school - of which his mother felt ashamed. In the initial meetings Paul's mother spoke for him, and relentlessly accused him, but was unable to consider the problem itself. The child psychotherapist arranged a few exploratory meetings with Paul on his own, while a colleague met with his mother.

In the two individual sessions, the child psychotherapist paid attention to this little boy (he was very undersized and immature): to his withdrawn and miserable manner, his silences, and the implications of his behaviour and difficult history (he was sent to live abroad with his grandparents for most of his life, and his father had died of drug-addiction one year previously). In the second meeting, feeling safe enough to risk the consequences and threats from his mother, he had asked if he could go and live in a children's home, and then talked about the beatings which he had kept hidden from all outsiders for two years.

In the light of follow-up long-term work, Paul's reference to the tattered bag was his way of talking about feeling maltreated and unsafe, showing how he was unable to hold onto his thoughts properly when he did not feel safely held in his mother's, or indeed anyone's mind. As his placement was still with a short-term foster mother, he found the uncertainty, upheavals and far-reaching implications hard to bear. The psychotherapy aimed to give Paul the opportunity to work through some of these feelings of distress. His anger was at times redirected onto the therapist, expressed partly by tearing up an appointment letter. He felt confused, guilty, uncertain, as well as, at times, a sense of loss.

Many of Paul's communications were non-verbal, indirect, or

symbolic. His reference, for example, to the bag full of holes was a symbolic expression of his feelings about himself and his mother, and were re-experienced with the therapist. With skilful listening, experience, and attention to her own emotional responses to the child, the therapist was gradually able to make sense of Paul's underlying feelings and feed them back to him in a way he could understand and hold inside himself. In time, Paul felt less like an inadequate and neglected 'bag full of holes' as he built up a sense of the therapist's ability to hold onto him in her mind over a period of time. He no longer needed to express his distress through the presenting symptom of stealing.

When do children need psychotherapy?

The kinds of problems children may demonstrate and which can be helpfully analysed within the safety of a therapeutic setting include: enuresis, encopresis, eating disorders, depression, sleep disturbances, over-clinging behaviour, aggression, school phobia, stealing, withdrawn behaviour, excessive masturbation, obsessional behaviour, poor ability to socialise, impaired learning or under-achievement, pseudo-maturity, fears, phobias, confusional states, being accident-prone, excessive escapes to a fantasy world and hyperactivity. The impact of chronic illness or physical or mental handicap, and the ways these affect their caregivers are probably further adequate reasons for the emotional understanding child psychotherapists can offer. Other adverse life events, such as lengthy hospitalisation, the death of someone close, lengthy separations, a seriously ill sibling or emotional environmental deprivation and abuse are pointers where, upon assessment, psychotherapy might be considered advisable.

Child psychotherapy, however, can only be carried out if the child's carers and support system (parents, foster parents or residential social workers) support the treatment. Generally, it is desirable that they participate in the treatment programme, perhaps by regularly seeing another professional who liaises with the child's therapist. If this is not possible, it can be all too easy for parents to undermine their child's treatment, however unintentionally, due to unacknowledged envy of the treatment the child is receiving. The minimum involvement with the carers would be regular review meetings with the child psychotherapist.

The child is viewed as a part of a wider unit. The option of family therapy may be ruled out if initial explorations reveal emotional difficulties in the child's own right or if significant family members are unavailable. However, the continual inter-relatedness and evolution of child and family or carers has to be facilitated alongside the child's development within the therapeutic relationship, so child psychotherapy is rarely carried out in isolation. While the detailed interaction must be confidential to facilitate trust and uncover layers with which other relationships need not concern themselves, the child needs to feel assured that the various adults in his or her life are working together.

Some treatments can be completed within a few weeks, if the problem is not deeply entrenched, but programmes usually last from at least a year up to several years. Frequency varies from regular once-weekly sessions to five times a week, and depends on availability of treatment, practical arrangements, the nature of the problem, and the child's ability to 'hold on' between sessions. For example, Emma, aged four, experienced the gaps between her weekly therapy sessions as an unbearable repetition of the feeling of being 'dropped' by previous foster placements which had broken down. When the therapy was increased to twice weekly sessions, Emma could begin to sustain hopefulness not only that there would be future sessions, but also that her therapist could bear and survive her aggressive attacks.

Improvements and developments in any therapy need to be consolidated, and this is done by repeating, for example, the experience of holiday breaks. This may arouse feelings of intolerable frustration, rage, manic defences, denial, sadness or loss. Time after time these reactions are re-experienced and brought to a level where they can be thought about and learnt from, so their sway over the child lessens. In this way, children gradually relinquish their need to excessively control the world or flee from it in their imagination, and take the often painful steps towards valuing the important people in their lives, accepting their dependence, and managing their infantile feelings.

Where is child psychotherapy practised?

Child psychotherapy is mainly practised in child guidance clinics, funded by either the health service, social services, education department or by a combination of these. Occasionally it is funded by a charity, or by the relatively recently created Child Psychotherapy Trust, which aims to promote the availability of child psychotherapy in the NHS. The service is also available in some hospitals or hospital child psychiatry departments as well as in some health centres, schools and counselling services. Some child psychotherapists work part-time in private practice.

Child psychotherapists also consult to other professionals who deal with children, such as nurses, hospital doctors, health visitors, nursery officers, child minders, teachers, GPs and social workers. Referrals come from all these professions, as well as from parents themselves. Consultative work is often preventive: problems can be dealt with before they become entrenched, or adults can simply be helped to think about management issues. This can be more effective and wide-reaching than when child psychotherapy is chosen as a 'last resort'.

Child psychotherapists also run small therapy groups for children of different ages and with different problems, such as adolescents, children who have been sexually abused and mothers and toddlers with eating problems. Group therapy is ideal for problems which can be shared with peers and, above all, are more rapidly unearthed in a group situation, where they can then be 'held' and interpreted by the group therapist.

In the hospital setting, child psychotherapists either work with children who have been referred to child psychiatry (with a similar population to child guidance clinics), or with children on the ward. This would include a wide range of situations, such as road traffic accident victims, cases of non-accidental injury, anorexia, attempted overdose cases, surgical and chronic conditions as well as children facing life-threatening illness. The aim is to address the children's concerns by offering anything from emotional 'first aid' to long-term intensive psychotherapy. It is well-documented that children tend to avoid expressing their anxieties to their parents for fear of upsetting them, and that parents similarly 'protect' their children by trying to be cheerful and avoiding the more serious implications of illness (Bluebond-Langner, 1978). This is where child psychotherapists (with the permission of the parents and, ideally, in conjunction with other members of a psychosocial team) help children to express their worries (Judd, 1989). Psychotherapy for children with cancer has been found to markedly decrease the frequency and severity of their emotional problems (Watson, 1983).

Working with parents

An important part of a child psychotherapist's work is with parents: not only regular reviews of the therapy and discussion of the parents' view of the child, but also work with parents in their own right. Pregnant women and mothers of very young babies may be in special need of a child psychotherapist's experience and understanding. Sarah, for example, a woman in her late twenties, sought help when she was experiencing negative feelings towards her unborn 'alien' baby and the changes to her body. Psychotherapy enabled her to understand how the unborn baby was imbued with her feelings of herself as an unwanted and unloved child. By the time of the birth, Sarah felt positive about her baby, and was able to mother him well, while continuing over several years to work in her therapy on her own 'infantile' feelings of worthlessness. In this way baby Ben was spared from having many of his mother's problems heaped upon him from birth, on top of the inevitable struggles of normal development.

There is a great need for the availability of child psychotherapy to spread beyond London. It is a cost-effective way of keeping children out of care, delinquency, and ultimately even prison or psychiatric hospital. Our children's future and accordingly that of the country as a whole would benefit if more services were available.

References
Bergmann, T. (1965) *Children in the Hospital*. International University Press, New York.
Judd, D. (1989) *Give Sorrow Words – Working with a Dying Child*. Free Association Books, London.
Watson, M. (1983) Psychological intervention with cancer patients: a review. *Psychological Medicine*, **13**, 839–46.

Bibliography

Bluebond-Langner, M. (1978) *The Private Worlds of Dying Children*. Princeton University Press, New Jersey.
 Illustrates clearly the way mutual protectiveness prevents patients and carers from communicating openly.
Boston, M. and Szur, R. (Eds) (1983) *Psychotherapy with Severely Deprived Children*. Routledge and Kegan Paul, London.
 Demonstrates how children previously considered unsuitable for psychotherapy have the capacity to respond to treatment.
Daws, D. and Boston, M. (Eds) (1977) *The Child Psychotherapist and Problems of Young People*. Wildwood House, London.
 A clear exposition, suitable for the lay reader, of many applications of child psychotherapy.

For more information and video contact:
The Child Psychotherapy Trust,
c/o TIHR,
Tavistock Centre,
120 Belsize Lane,
London NW3 5BA.
Tel: 071-433 3867.

Careers leaflet available from:
The Association of Child Psychotherapists,
Burgh House,
New End Square,
London NW3 1LT.
Tel: 071-794 8881.

Adolescence:
Health Concerns

21

Altered body image in anorexia nervosa

Stephanie J. Wright
Third year Student Nurse, Royal Devon and Exeter Hospital, Exeter

Contrary to the common belief, anorexia is not a modern disease; it has in fact been with us at least since the Victorian era, when it was documented and illustrated. Girls were noted to refuse food or dispose of it by various methods (appropriately vague for the proper Victorian society); they became thin, wore voluminous clothing and scraped their hair back from their faces to show their 'slimness'. The picture is remarkably consistent with the characteristics displayed by many anorexics today.

A disease of the west

As western society has become more affluent, with food available to refuse, anorexia nervosa has become increasingly well documented as a disease of the western world; only in places with a surplus of food do people *decide* to starve themselves to the edge of death. Previously the illness had been seen as a set of physical signs and symptoms sparked off by rather simplistic reasons for the girl's (women outnumber men, although the number of male anorexics is now rising) initial decision to stop eating. Such reasons may include: a method of getting back at one's mother; a way of objecting to the permissive role; a rejection of female (or male) sexuality; an attempt at committing slow suicide.

It is now recognised that although these may be influencing factors in the initial decision, they are by no means the sole reason, and to reduce the illness thus is to over simplify it beyond recognition. From this picture, a cure should be an easy task of reversing one warped way of thinking; I hope to illustrate that this is very far from the truth, and indicate the conceptual changes which the anorexic undergoes. The anorexic will be referred to as 'she', female sufferers being more common, but it is recognised that men have equal problems when they become anorexic.

Changes in behaviour

The anorexic's behaviour changes as the illness progresses and so do the reasons for refusing to eat. The psychological problems follow as predictable a pattern as the physical process. This is best illustrated by a classic American study in which a group of soldiers were compared to a group of well educated middle class girls in the way they might respond to the anorexic's diet, which also describes the disease process.

For six months the soldiers were kept on a diet of 1,572 calories per day, a level at which most men would begin to lose weight. As time went on the soldiers became more preoccupied with food, in fact they read cookery books in preference to anything else. On shopping trips they even bought kitchen utensils although they had no use for them and on the whole were quite unable to explain such actions.

Their emotional behaviour also underwent considerable change, as they became increasingly antisocial and irritable. They became further depressed and their interest in sex diminished rapidly. During this time the soldiers kept detailed records of how they felt and the emotional changes they underwent. They were immensely self-critical, feeling disgust and self-loathing, and described a feeling of 'deep, dark depression'. They felt low, bad, full of guilt and self-hatred and their records were full of accounts of episodes of uncontrolled eating, where they would gorge themselves and then force themselves to vomit. The soldiers also turned to shoplifting and petty theft, and became very restless and hyperactive. It also became increasingly difficult to talk to the soldiers and the researchers frequently felt that they were being lied to.

This strange behaviour is reported as psychopathy of the person suffering from anorexia nervosa and it is now believed that a progressive reduction in food leads to a steady decline in the suffer's intellectual capacity. This can be explained by looking at the hemispheres of the brain, where the highest functions of reason and abstract thought take place. There is a maze of potential, rather than specific, pathways of neural activity and if these are disturbed, such as by starvation, higher functions are impaired. The decrease in the mental capacity of the soldiers showed in three ways: first, their selfishness, withdrawal from social situations and a decreased interest in sex. Second, their remaining mental capacity was concentrated on food, and third, their thought processes became more polarised with only the extremes of good or bad left open to them.

As anorexics become more self-centred the problems of the world diminish and they see things 'clearly' through a calm detachment. Everything is seen in relation to food, and success relates to the anorexic's ability to control her eating.

Distorted sense of appearance

The typical anorexic is a perfectionist, achievement-orientated young woman (13-25 years old) who seeks to rule her life by controlling her body. Even as she becomes dangerously emaciated, the distorted sense of her own appearance tells her that she is grotesquely fat. (AJN, 1984). Despite having "everything to live for" and appearing confident and in control of her life, the anorexic (or potential anorexic) only feels to be in command of the situation when she has a vice-like grip on her dietary intake. It is difficult for non-anorexics to comprehend but she sees starvation as a positive thing, her aim is to be thin and starvation helps her achieve this. By now her thought processes are sufficiently distorted as to make her unaware of her dangerous state of health, and her own self perception makes her see herself as revoltingly obese and some form of grotesque 'freak'. It is now most apparent that the anorexic's body image is grossly distorted.

When a person's body weight falls well below what it may naturally be expected to be, severe communication problems develop, leading to classic anorexic perception and behaviour. This is reversed if the weight begins to increase but while parents and other people looking after her may find this physical improvement very rewarding, it is a crisis for the anorexic. If she gains a viable body weight, communication becomes easier, menstruation returns and hyperactivity is not so apparent, but she suffers from a drop in self esteem, as well as depression and anxiety, she becomes very sensitive to the demands of others and finds it almost impossible to make even minor decisions.

As one anorexic put it '(Self-starvation) is exchanging confusion, conflict and feelings of failure for a sense of calm clarity and feelings of success'. (Llewellyn-Jones and Abraham, 1984).

By returning her to normal methods of eating, one is robbing the anorexic of her only feelings of success and sometimes even sanity but once she discovers methods of weight removal, such as self induced vomiting and/or laxative abuse, she has a new found confidence. She can eat to appease her worried parents while maintaining her concept of her body image, safe in the knowledge that she can lose weight when she requires. Her weight will still fluctuate, but will tend to be within a specific range, rather than from very wild extremes. The anorexic can even show

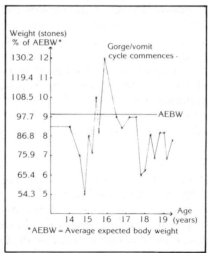

Figure 1. Fluctuations in weight gained and lost in the anorexic.

her frantic parents that she has 'put on' weight, knowing that she can vomit it afterwards. (Figure 1).

Anorexics fail to realise that this behaviour actually makes it more likely that they will continue to starve themselves. They feel that to achieve 'model' status they must be as 'slim' as a model (ie underweight); also the detached feeling accompanying the illness is taken as a positive thing. They feel it puts them more 'in touch' with themselves and clears the mind so they can concentrate on important things in their lives. This is known as polarised thinking; as the illness progresses, it leaves fewer and fewer options, ending only with extremes of 'good' and 'bad'.

At the good extreme is the preferred image of herself. To keep this, and hence her self-esteem and morale, requires intense concentration. Failure to maintain an adequate control has profound implications on her perceived body image which will swing to the bad extreme.

Inability to compromise

The intransigence of the anorexic's thought processes related to her own image is reflected quite well in the behaviour of political hunger strikers. As they deteriorate physically, their demands become more rigid; the downwards spiral of their mental capacity makes them unable to cope with the complex abstracts involved in compromise, so the mental consequences of self starvation appear to illustrate superhuman self sacrifice and a devotion to cause. This is the 'whirlpool effect' (Slade, 1984); the anorexic's condition spirals downwards, even though the original reason for her behaviour may no longer apply, so she continues starving herself for different reasons to those that made her start.

Drawing together all these facts relating to the psychological behaviour of the anorexic illustrates that to have any therapeutic relationship at all, one must not just attempt to force the body weight up, as this will only serve to alienate the girl and destroy any previous relationship formed.

Merely dealing in weight gain will leave the girl worse than before as she will be depressed and worthless in her own eyes. In any case, the severe anorexic will see herself as doing well at six stone 13 pounds, but obese at seven stone because of the limited and extreme categories into which she falls. She also deals with people's comments in an extreme way; 'You look well today', will be interpreted as 'You look horribly fat' and protestations to the contrary will only convince her further.

Split personality

The anorexic feels almost to have a split personality, one chaotic and full of failure (eating) and the other successful and well controlled (starvation). The only tragedy of this 'equilibrium' is that the maintenance of an extreme weight is not possible and the girl will either have to undergo the humiliation of outside intervention or will lose the battle to her 'bad' self and have internal humiliation; either way, there is no escape.

Bargaining with the girl may be the only way to gain any progress in this situation. By agreeing to try to maintain her weight at 70 per cent of average expected body weight, the anorexic can be spared the humiliation of in-patient admission, and she can remain in control without having to undergo the trauma of buying larger clothing. She will also have a biologically safe body weight, although to the 'normal' person she will still look rather thin.

The current death rate from complications relating to anorexia nervosa in Britain is approximately four per cent. Whilst this is a very small number the number of upwardly mobile, ambitious and young people (although these characteristics are not universal) in whom it causes increasing debility appears to be growing. In order to effect a 'cure' for these people, those who look after them must understand the perceptual changes they experience to give them the empathy required to do this.

References
AJN (1984) Avoiding the power struggle. *American Journal of Nursing*, Editorial, **84**, 1, 30–35.
Llewellyn Jones, D. and Abraham, S. (1984) Eating Disorders: the Facts. OUP, Oxford.
Slade, R. (1984) The Anorexia Nervosa Reference Book. Harper and Row, London.

Bibliography
Aniskowitz, S. (1984) Anorexia Nervosa, *Nursing Mirror*, **158**, 15, 42–43.
Gibson, E. (1983) Babytalk. *Nursing Times*, **79**, 7, 64.
Solzhenitzyn, A. (1963) A Day in the Life of Ivan Denisovitch. Gollanz, London.

Useful address
Anorexic Aid, The Priory Centre, 11 Priory Road, High Wycombe, Bucks. They offer support and advice to sufferers of anorexia and bulimia.

22

Anorexia bulimia

Jo S. Burns, RMN
Staff Nurse, Pastures Hospital, Derby

The typical bulimia sufferer will not be thin and undernourished, refusing all food; she will probably be within her normal weight range for her height but a few pounds below her ideal weight. She has insight into her problem/behaviour and is therefore receptive to treatment (Herzog and Copeland, 1985). She knows exactly what she is doing and may even be able to explain some of the reasons. As treatment progresses, many more causes or contributory factors are discovered and brought out into the open. The feelings that initiate the behaviour are overwhelming and impossible to control. ''Unlike anorexic patients, bulimics experience a deep sense of shame and are aware of the possible consequences of their behaviour, but also fear the loss of controlling their eating'' (Balaa and Drossman, 1985).

Paulette Maisner, who runs the Maisner Centre of Eating Disorders in Brighton feels that people who 'give' a lot of themselves emotionally and physically are more likely to suffer from eating disorders, and that nurses are therefore more susceptible to developing them (Maisner, 1985).

Bulimia sufferers are generally older than those who suffer from anorexia nervosa, ranging in age between 18 and 40. Approximately 50 per cent of bulimia sufferers will have a history of anorexia nervosa. An average of 13.7 per cent of females will be lifetime sufferers of anorexia bulimia. There are far fewer male sufferers.

Pattern of behaviour
An individual with anorexia feels that he/she has a split personality: ''one chaotic and full of failure (eating) and the other is successful and well-controlled (starvation)'' (Wright, 1986).

A similar situation occurs with the bulimia sufferer. One half of her has an overwhelming desire to be slim, to cope, to be accepted, to control herself and her life, while the other has to binge and vomit to maintain the acceptable part of her. To be slim she will eat very little, almost to the point of starvation, believing that she is in control and therefore acceptable because she is slim. Emotionally she will appear flat, calm, depressed and even abrupt. Depressive symptoms are common in anorexia nervosa and bulimia. In one study, 50 per cent of anorexic patients and more than 20 per cent of bulimia patients met criteria for a major depressive disorder (Herzog and Copeland, 1985). This behaviour occurs because she is trying to please an important person in her life, who is likely to have a dominant, successful, unemotional character. It may be a parent, husband or wife, boyfriend or girlfriend — someone from whom the bulimia sufferer requires approval which she hopes will ultimately lead to 'love' and/or appreciation. Feelings of inadequacy, passivity, and a tendency to look to men for confirmation of their sense of worth have all been reported to characterise these patients (Balaa and Drossman, 1985). Indeed, the need to be loved and accepted, to be correct may be the root of the problem.

It can be seen that the bulimia sufferer also has two conflicting aspects to her personality, is less influenced to be slim by media pressure but is driven by a deep need for love and affection.

Self-hate

This unhappy but controlled personality will be most disturbed by the very person she aims to please, or any stressful situation or event that undermines her control over her emotions and eating. Despite all efforts the individual with bulimia is usually unable to make this dominant, successful person happy. Something will always be at fault, and whenever the dominant person expresses disapproval of her, she will experience an overwhelming feeling of disgust and self hate. She thinks that the person she most wants to approve of her thinks she is disgusting, vile, obese, stupid and so on and that he or she is right. At this point she turns to food.

Binging, consuming amazing quantities of food; loaves of bread; six Mars bars; three or four packets of biscuits; pounds of cheese; bacon; sausages; cakes; more chocolate; potatoes — clarifies this disgust. It is almost an act of violence, fuelled by anger against the person whose approval she wanted, and supported by anger and hatred for herself. The sufferer must hide her anger towards the dominant person, for fear he might leave her, then she would never have his approval, or receive his love and affection. So she eats and abuses herself, going to great lengths to acquire all the food necessary for a full scale binge. She may go to the supermarket, buy enough for an army, explaining to the cashier that it is for a large family, then go home and eat as much of it as possible, she may eat all the food in the house, or even resort to stealing. Throughout this process she feels extremely guilty but the tremendous desire for food puts her in a frenzy.

Consolation

The binge will be held guiltily, in secret and must not on any account be interrupted so may take place during the night. It brings a transient consolation for a deep sadness and dissatisfaction. The sufferer needs warmth and comfort and will turn to food to acquire it — just as some people may turn to casual sex. For the bulimia sufferer sexual contact is too adult and too threatening. To attempt physical consolation with another person would provide the opportunity for further rejection.

Vomiting

The vomiting is induced so that this consolation can be enjoyed without a gain in weight and to make room for further binging. With practice, automatic, self-induced vomiting can be achieved, making the whole process considerably easier. The realisation that vomiting is a solution to the problem of how to eat as much as you like but still be slim ensures that self-induced vomiting continues.

Repeated vomiting is physically harmful as well as habit forming. Unchecked, it may cause metabolic disorders, weakness, kidney failure, tachycardia, tetany, low blood pressure, fluid retention, dental erosion and mouth ulcers. Occasionally the parotid glands become swollen (parotitis) causing the neck and cheeks to enlarge as in mumps.

Some patients use laxatives instead of, or with, vomiting. Purgative abuse may produce diarrhoea or constipation and loss of bowel tone.

After the sufferer has been consoled by the food and her guilt about how much she has consumed alleviated by vomiting or purging, she may feel ashamed of the episode but suppresses it and compensates by practically starving herself and being 'in control' again – until the next time.

Care approach

Help and treatment for a bulimia sufferer might begin with an in depth assessment interview lasting for about an hour or more when information about past life; childhood; present home situation; family relationships, past and present; opinions of self and feelings could be gathered, as these factors could be significant in developing an understanding of the origins of the client's particular problems. It can also contribute to building up a good working relationship between client and nurse.

The client would be asked to keep a diary of all her food intake, including binges, so that the extent of the eating disorder might be assessed. After a week or two with the assessment made, the client would be asked to stop using the diary to take the emphasis off food and to not reinforce the problem.

A diet would be devised consisting of foods that the client feels that she could enjoy regularly. Not a weight increasing diet, but low fat, high energy foods such as bread, potatoes and rice, and healthy amounts of protein, fruit and vegetables. Moderate amounts of biscuits, sweets, yoghurts and puddings could be encouraged if the client desired and remembered them as normal.

At first the client should be weighed once a week with the aim of maintaining a stable weight with which both client and therapist are happy. She should also be encouraged to have an occupation to divert her mind from food, her problems and the treatment. Ideally it should be a hobby that the client enjoys and does well, to boost her self-esteem and assist treatment. After the initial assessment, regular daily sessions of a set length could be arranged.

Involvement

During the regular sessions the client could discuss any worries she may have about her treatment. She may suggest alterations or offer further information which she feels may be significant. Her involvement would be very important. Both client and therapist should look for factors which may precipitate binges. A chart to record observations might be useful.

The daily sessions could be used to educate the client about how life threatening her behaviour is. It should be explained how abuse of laxatives and diuretics causes electrolyte inbalance and therefore tachycardia, low blood pressure, fluid retention and possibly finger oedema. How excessive vomiting can cause dental erosion, mouth ulcers and parotitis. The importance of a regular balanced diet to ensure the body receives all the vitamins and nutrients it requires should also be explained.

Family counselling

Family counselling might be suggested to discuss any problems within the family and how they possibly contribute to the client's condition. If improvement is steady, the number of sessions should be reduced to three a week, then two, then one a week, to reduce the client's dependence on the therapist. At this point, individual or group psychotherapy might be an option, but as Herzog and Copeland state: "No controlled studies on the efficiency of psychodynamic psychotherapy, group therapy, or family therapy in eating disorders are available" (Herzog and Copeland, 1985). When both the client and therapist feel confident, the client should be discharged and referred to the community team for follow up, which may involve regular weekly visits and referral to self help groups or to a day centre.

Prognosis

As yet no statistics are available about success or reversal rates. However, Herzog and Copeland state that "although bulimia patients are more motivated to seek treatment, they frequently have a low frustration tolerance and may have difficulty tolerating therapeutic situations that do not produce immediate relief of symptoms." Prognosis is therefore at best uncertain.

References

Balaa and Drossman (1985) Anorexia nervosa and bilimia: The eating disorders. *Disease a Month*, 3, 6.

Chudley, P. (1986) Unhealthy obsession. *Nursing Times*, **82**, 50.

Herzog and Copeland (1985) Eating disorders, *New England Journal of Medicine*, **313**, 5, 295–303.

Savage, S. and Biley, F. (1984) Bulimia nervosa, *Nursing Times*, **80**, 43.

Wright, S.J. (1986) Altered body image in anorexia nervosa. *The Professional Nurse*, **1**, 10, 260-2.

23

Why do adolescents smoke?

ALISON STEWART, RGN, RM, RHV, MSc
Research Midwife, Bristol Maternity Hospital

JUDY ORME, BSc
Research Assistant, International Centre for Child Studies

Smoking is a controversial subject, at times arousing emotions and reactions similar to those engendered by politics and religion. Even with the proven associated health hazards people continue to smoke. In 1986 35 per cent of men and 31 per cent of women smoked in the UK (OPCS Monitor, 1988). While smokers are now a minority of the population, the habit is still a major preventable cause of premature death. As a result, with regard to health issues the habit maintains a high profile in the public awareness. Action against smoking has been two-fold: helping existing smokers to stop (Kendall, 1986), and preventing the habit becoming established. Preventive education means focusing on children, and realising smoking in childhood and adolescence is widespread.

Adolescent smoking

A national survey of smoking, conducted by the Office of Population Census and Surveys (OPCS), among secondary school children in England and Wales in 1986, revealed that between 6–10 per cent smoked regularly (>1 cigarette per week) compared with 13 per cent in 1984. More than half claimed to have never smoked (Goddard, 1989). This apparent downward trend is encouraging, but the information that one in 10 children smokes regularly indicates the potential health risks accruing in this generation. It is estimated that 40 times more young men who are regular smokers will die as a consequence of smoking than will die in road traffic accidents (Peto, 1980). Recognising the problem entails devising some action to try and reduce this hazard as far as possible, for example formulating anti-smoking material. The aim must ultimately be to try and ensure that children neither 'drift' into smoking, nor are coerced into it: at best it should be an informed choice.

Models of smoking

Exponents from various disciplines have tried to create models to explain why people smoke. These have had psychological, psychosocial, pharmacological and genetic bases. However, it remains difficult to incorporate the different elements into a comprehensive model which will apply to all individuals. The work of developmental theorists is of considerable use in trying to understand this behaviour. Smoking is then seen as a process with different stages such as preparation, initiation, establishment and maintenance.

Who is smoking?

The 1988 OPCS survey reported that amongst secondary schoolchildren, the prevalence of cigarette smoking remained higher among girls than boys (Goddard, 1989). However, for both sexes there was a downward trend in numbers smoking compared to surveys in 1984 and 1986. Whilst fewer boys than girls were regularly or occasionally smoking in 1988, more boys had actually tried and then not pursued the habit. Slightly more girls than boys reported having given up smoking.The sex differentiated smoking behaviour suggests different factors are involved in the decision to smoke. Girls may be more conscious of using cigarettes to try and regulate their weight or to emulate a 'cool', sexually attractive woman. Boys may be more concerned with limitations smoking may place on athletic prowess.

Among 11-16 year-olds, as age increases, the proportion of never-smokers decreases, with regular smoking being most prevalent in the older age groups of 14-16 years. In the Brigantia survey (Charlton, 1984a) of 16,000 nine to 19-year-olds of those having tried a cigarette, one per cent claimed to have had a puff of a cigarette by the age of four.

Influences

Family   Much childhood social learning occurs in the home as children copy other members of the family. In the Brigantia survey, children were twice as likely to be smokers if their parents smoked. The effects of sibling smoking behaviour are even more marked. In the OPCS 1988 survey, 26% of pupils with a sibling who smoked were regular smokers themselves compared to only 5% with a non-smoking sibling. Which indicates that a non-smoking sibling in the home may reduce the chances of a pupil becoming a regular smoker (Goddard, 1989).

Peers   Other studies have concentrated on the effects of peer group pressure. Bewley and Bland (1977) in a study of 491 schoolchildren aged 10-10½ found that 76 per cent of smokers had friends who smoked compared to 36 per cent of non-smokers. Inevitably, friends can exert considerable influence and act as or sources of supply.

School   The milieu provided at school with curriculum teaching, teacher/pupil example and relations of different peer groups, can act as a stimulus or a deterrent on becoming a smoker. Varying rates of smoking can occur between different types of school in the same geographical area (Banks et al, 1978). In view of the instability of many home situations, schools may be a major influence, representing a constant feature in a changing childhood. Nash (1987) reported that 14-

16 year-olds appeared to smoke partly for the pleasure of rebelling against school authority. Bewley and Bland (1977) found that both children's self-ratings and those of teachers assessed non-smokers as academically better. This may be due to time taken smoking – or obtaining income for it – having a detrimental effect on school performance or due to low-achievers boosting their morale by smoking.

Adolescence is commonly associated with a period of crisis and confusion as the individual changes from a child to an adult. The dissonance our society creates in terms of employment prospects, Youth Training Schemes, sexual freedom and so on heightens teenagers' sense of their anomalous position. Self-esteem and confidence may be low, and smoking may raise morale and reduce tension.

As a smoker
Each adolescent's perception of the effects of smoking will depend on how smoking is learned to be associated with changes in physical/mental states. These changes can then be labelled as pleasant or aversive and the example of family and friends can contribute to this.

Intention to give up
Some adolescents in the 1988 OPCS survey who were not currently smoking anticipated that they would smoke before leaving school. Grouped by current smoking status, this included never-smokers (4%), tried smoking once (10%) and used to smoke (29%). The fact that very few of these same pupils thought that they would become regular smokers suggests the importance of tobacco usage in school culture; a function which may change when leaving school. Regular smokers are more likely to anticipate continuing smoking beyond school years (63%). Adolescence is a time in which young people try out different roles, images and behaviours.

Health
The detrimental consequences of smoking on health are well documented and effects may occur very early in a smoker's life. In children aged 10-12½ years, respiratory symptoms (eg coughs) correlated with smoking. Regular smokers reported more symptoms than occasional smokers, who reported more than never-smokers (Bewley and Bland, 1976). Future mortality and morbidity effects appear to be increased when smoking starts before the age of 15 years (Hammond, 1966). Of particular current concern are the potential health risks of girls smoking, and also using the contraceptive pill.

Leisure
Banks et al (1978), found smokers were more likely to go to a youth club, go round with a group of their own age and have a friend of the opposite sex, rather than stay at home reading. Obviously, activities create opportunities to experiment and to conform to the existing peer culture.

Media and advertising

Television advertising of cigarettes was banned in 1965, but tobacco companies now use subtle pressures such as sports sponsorship to obtain viewing time exposure to brand names. Films and soap-operas can provide both negative and positive images of smoking through heroes and anti-heroes, which may exert a counter pressure to attempts to inform children of the risks of smoking. The tobacco industry tries to justify poster advertising by claiming they may increase brand awareness and encourage smokers to change to lower tar cigarettes. However, it has been argued that the advertisements contain minimal information and may also influence non-smokers (Chapman, 1985).

Beliefs about smoking

Knowledge about smoking comes from numerous sources, in particular, significant others, such as the family, and may determine children's smoking behaviour. For example, if all the family and friends smoke, smoking may appear a natural activity like eating and sleeping. Charlton (1984b) found that smokers associated 'calms nerves' with smoking, while never-smokers and ex-smokers associated negative aspects of the behaviour such as it being a waste of money and smelly. However, knowledge is not always applied to self. A sample of 16-17 year-olds revealed more regular smokers than non-smokers associated cigarettes with the word 'cancer'. They also exhibited a well developed awareness of the health risks yet continued to smoke (Charlton, 1982). This might suggest that the information of a long-term risk has little impact on short-term decisions to smoke – the risk is not perceived as 'real'.

Health education

The extent to which children are exposed to health education varies between schools. In the OPCS 1986 survey, 42 per cent of secondary school children had received a lesson on smoking in the previous year (Goddard and Ikin, 1987), whereas this had risen to 52% in 1988 (Goddard, 1989). The percentage was lowest among first-years and highest among fifth-years, so many of the early smokers are not being reached in time. Subjects such as health and hygiene received a larger coverage than emotive issues like smoking and alcohol (Goddard, 1989).

The nurse's role

Nurses have a major role in combating adolescent smoking. The aim must be three-fold: discourage individuals starting or continuing; provide realistic, understandable information about the risks, so that those smoking are making an informed choice, and provide sufficient support for those who choose to give up smoking.

In schools   School nurses and health visitors have extended their role beyond routine screening examinations to involvement in the provision of curriculum health education. It is important to ensure that smoking is not neglected in favour of more topical areas such as AIDS or more neutral ones such as diet and hygiene. Since many children try smoking at an early age, discussions about smoking may be appropriate even at early primary school age. It is important to appreciate the diversity of influences for adolescents and children smoking. Formal lectures may be of limited value, since they may not have the scope to confront all the erroneous beliefs which individual smokers may hold such as 'I smoke to be slim', and 'cancer can be cured'. Group discussions using a starting strategy of asking participants what they think/believe about the subject can be invaluable, and are as relevant for non-smokers as smokers. Ideas for presentations of material include:

- Group discussions on any issue related to smoking. Many programmes in the USA have sought to explore adolescents' self-perceptions and support their self-esteem to enable them to withstand social pressures to conform and smoke.
- Lectures on health risks, physiology of smoking, economic and social aspects of the habit.
- Using the current teaching aids/courses, GCSE has several useful active learning books and there are various TV broadcasts for schools.
- Linking in with national anti-smoking awareness campaigns such as the annual National No-Smoking Day.

Increasing emphasis is being placed on active learner participation and as nurses we need to consider how to use this type of teaching method effectively to communicate our message.

The example of individuals such as teachers and nurses can contribute to the decision to smoke. To discourage children from smoking and then be seen smoking negates the whole message. We need to consider our behaviour and its influence on others in contact with children, eg encouraging schools to adopt a non-smoking policy for staff.

Action in the family   Nurses in any specialty can advise adults about the injurious effects of smoking and the effect parental influence has on children's habits. Future parents may therefore be inculcated with more responsible attitudes towards their children's health.

The primary care team   Nurses working in treatment rooms or offering family planning services can discuss smoking on an individual basis as part of a check-up. In a one-to-one discussion it may be possible to provide specific incentives to an adolescent to give up or not take up smoking. It is particularly important for family planning nurses to try to discover the 'true' smoking habits of teenagers seeking contraception and advise them on the risks of choosing to take the Pill and smoke.

Action in society   This may involve all nurses with measures such as campaigning for the Government to ban all forms of tobacco advertisements and discourage consumption with increased added tax on cigarettes. Nurses may also be involved in activities with young people such as Guides, Scouts and church clubs, which may provide the opportunity of approaching the subject of smoking in a more social setting than classrooms or surgeries.

Since many adolescents say they intend to stop smoking, there is a need for considerable support and encouragement to help them do so. Many smokers comment that a major problem in giving up is not succumbing to the craving, often when they have apparently successfully stopped. When advising smokers to stop, nurses must consider the feasibility of either setting up counselling/support groups or at least putting the individual in contact with a pre-existing one.

References
Banks, M.H. et al (1978) Long-term study of smoking by secondary school children. *Arch. of Dis. in Childhood*, **53,** 12–19.
Bewley, B.R. and Bland, J.M. (1976) Smoking and respiratory symptoms in two groups of schoolchildren. *Preventive Medicine*, **5,** 63–69.
Bewley, B.R. and Bland, J.M. (1977) Academic performance and social factors related to cigarette smoking by school children. *British Journal of Preventive and Social Medicine*, **31,** 18–24.
Charlton, A. (1982) Lung Cancer: the ultimate smoking deterrent for young people. *Journal of the IHE*, **20,** 2, 5–15.
Charlton, A. (1984a) The Brigantia smoking survey: a general review. In: *Public Education about Cancer*, UICC Technical Report Series: 77, 92–102.
Charlton, A. (1984b) Children's opinions about smoking. *Jnl. RCGP*, **3,** 483-87.
Chapman, S. (1985) Cigarette advertising and smoking: a review of the evidence. In: *Smoking out the Barons 1986*. John Wiley, London.
Goddard, E. (1989) *Smoking among secondary schoolchildren in England, 1988*. HMSO, London.
Goddard, E. and Ikin, C. (1987) *Smoking among secondary schoolchildren in 1986*. HMSO, London.
Hammond, E.C. (1966) Smoking in relation to death rates of one million men and women. *National Cancer Institute Monograph*, **19,** 127.
Kendall, S. (1986) Helping people to stop smoking. *The Professional Nurse*, **1,** 120–23.
Nash, J. (1987). Sparking up – smoking and style in school. *Health Ed. Jnl.* **46,** 152-55. OPCS Monitor Cigarette Smoking: 1972 to 1986, SS 88/1 9/2/88.
Peto, R. (1980) Possible ways of explaining the quantitative dangers of smoking. *Health Ed. Jnl.*, **39,** 2, 45-6.

Bibliography
Jacobsen, B. (1986) Beating the Ladykillers. Pluto Press, London.
    A broad range of issues including feminist aspects and Third World involvement.

Useful addresses
Leaflets and Factsheets produced by ASH 75p for a set of eight factsheets on health aspects and economics of smoking. Margaret Pyke House, 27–35 Mortimer Street, London W1N 7RJ.
Information sheet by GASP, 37 Stokes Croft, Bristol BS1 3PY. Useful, up-to-date information with some relevance to adolescent issues.

Acknowledgement
To Cancer Research Campaign for funding to undertake the analysis of Youthscan data with reference to smoking. It is hoped that the results from the survey of the third national cohort (16,000 babies born in 1970) at the age of 16 years, will provide information on some of the issues discussed in this article.

24

Malignant melanoma: mole watching and the adolescent

Pauline J. Perkins, BSc (Hons), RGN, ONC, RM Dip N
Lecturer in Surgical Nursing, University of Southampton

Malignant melanoma is now considered to be a significant health problem in the white adult population. In certain European countries the incidence of this disease is doubling every 10 – 15 years. During 1988, 3,000 new cases were reported in England and Wales. Current overall figures for the UK suggest only 65% of patients with melanoma will survive 5 years (MacKie, 1989).

Melanoma is not considered a disease of childhood. However, increasing evidence suggest that excessive childhood sun exposure is an important factor in its aetiology (Hurwitz, 1988; Lew *et al.*, 1983). Other studies support this in warning that painful blistering sunburns in childhood and adolescence are associated with an increased risk (Rhodes *et al.*, 1987; Green, 1984). Repeated exposure to high intensity solar ultraviolet radiation, gender, host pigmentation and reaction to sunlight have all been identified as contributing factors in the aetiology of melanoma (Dubin *et al.*, 1986). In view of this somewhat alarming evidence it may be useful to gain a better understanding of the disease and possible preventive strategies which may be directed towards adolescents.

What is malignant melanoma?

Malignant melanoma is the most serious, and often fatal, form of skin cancer which commonly arises in a naevus (mole) or appears as a new lesion on the skin. It involves the pigment producing cells (melanocytes) of the skin and has the ability to spread to other organs of the body.

There are four main types of malignant melanoma:
- superficial spreading melanoma
- modular melanomas
- acral melanomas
- lentigo maligna melanomas

The most common being superficial spreading melanoma which characteristically has a lateral growth phase prior to an invasive growth phase.

Nodular melanomas represent approximately 20–25% of all melanomas but carry a poorer prognosis for two reasons. Firstly, nodular melanomas are difficult to recognise clinically, even to an expert eye. Secondly, the invasive growth phase starts immediately which makes it a rapidly growing tumour with increased chance of secondary spread.

The remaining two types of melanoma are acral and lentigo maligna melanoma. Acral melanomas are seen on the palms and soles but may also include subungual tumours which often are amelanotic in nature. Lentigo maligna is a clinically benign pigmented lesion which may be present on sun-exposed areas of skin for many years. The term lentigo maligna melanoma is used when the lesion becomes an invasive malignant tumour.

Survival rates

Unfortunately, the five year survival rates in the UK for melanoma are lower than in any other country, and prognosis appears to be dependent upon tumour thickness (Breslow, 1970). Tumours less than 0.78mm thick are regarded as potentially curable and carry an excellent prognosis. Where Breslow's thickness is reported to be greater than 1.5mm, a good prognosis is less certain.

If left untreated, melanoma has the capability of metastasising to other organs in the body via the circulatory and lymphatic systems. This characteristic differentiates melanoma from the more common, less serious forms of skin cancer, basal cell carcinoma and squamous cell carcinoma where local spread is usual.

Therefore, it is vital melanoma is recognised and excised at an early stage in its development. Thin non-invasive tumours are effectively treated with conservative surgery. Late stage melanoma, where there is evidence of widespread secondary deposits, carries a far poorer prognosis. Treatments for late stage disease such as radiotherapy, chemotherapy, bio-immunotherapy and laser surgery, as yet offer no curative outcomes and are purely palliative in nature.

Melanoma is relatively rare, accounting for only 3% of all primary cutaneous malignancies. It is however responsible for two thirds of the deaths attributable to skin cancer. Another important aspect of the epidemiology of this disease concerns the number of young adults affected, which may be due to the amount of sun exposure during the first 20 years of life. Of melanoma cases 22% occur in people aged less than 40, whereas only 4% of all malignant neoplasms occur in this age group. Melanoma is the fourth commonest cancer in women aged between 15 and 34 years. It is the seventh commonest cancer in men.

Prevention of melanoma

Preventive measures which may be taken in avoiding any disease may be classified as primary, secondary and tertiary and are grouped according to the stage of disease at which they are intended to have their effect (Muir-Gray and Fowler, 1984).

Tertiary prevention

Traditionally nurses have been involved in tertiary prevention of melanoma. This can be interpreted as nursing intervention which involves care, treatment and rehabilitation of a person with symptomatic disease. Frequently this involves the holistic care of the dying patient, or the care and rehabilitation of the cancer patient in remission.

As melanoma is extremely rare in childhood and adolescence, primary and secondary preventive measures are more appropriate and may be successfully utilized by nurses in their role as health educator.

Primary prevention

The main aim in primary prevention is complete avoidance of disease. This is particularly pertinent here as the main target populations in any primary prevention strategy are children, adolescents and their parents. Examples of primary preventive measures are fluoridation, immunisation, provision of vitamin supplements and health education. In preventing malignant melanoma, health education is the cornerstone to any preventive strategy.

Health education programme   Since the main controllable causal factor of melanoma is sun exposure a major step forward in preventing this disease is the implementation of health education programmes in schools, on the dangers of excessive sun exposure. During 1990, education programmes designed specifically for adolescents (*Sun Cool*, Imperial Cancer Research Fund) and primary school children (*Monty Mole's Marvellous Mission*, Wessex Cancer Trust), were developed and successfully implemented as local pilot studies. These studies have generated much interest in furthering the development of health education programmes throughout the UK.

There appears to be a general acceptance in recent years that health promotion during childhood and adolescence profoundly influences the physical and psychosocial development of the child and ultimately of the young adult. This would be one of the main aims in any primary prevention programme for skin cancer. Current attitudes, beliefs and behaviours regarding sunshine may be a contributing factor to the increasing incidence of melanoma over recent years. Sunshine generates feelings of psychological and physical wellbeing. This helps in understanding why adolescents and young adults actively encourage, and demonstrate 'sunseeking' behaviours. The development of an all over tan is fashionable and described as attractive. The present argument is whether it is really healthy. Here lies the fundamental problem in delivering a health education programme to adolescents as socialisation processes are deeply influential in determining behaviours.

Socialisation, behaviour and the adolescent   White (1977) describes socialisation as more than just formal education. It includes attitude and value formation. Behaviours, habits and skills are learned during the process of socialisation via the family initially, then through other agencies such as schools, peer groups and the mass media. Adolescents are particularly influenced by peers and the general media. This may have advantages and disadvantages regarding the success of health education messages on skin cancer and the dangers of sunlight.

An individual's desire to have a tan may be strongly influenced by peers and fashion, therefore any health education message should allow one to enjoy the benefits of fine weather yet avoid melanoma and premature aging. One positive approach is the suggestion of slight behaviour modification: *avoid burning*, rather than denying time in the sun which is often viewed as unacceptable.

Environmental issues feature strongly in any school curriculum. Children and adolescents are increasingly more concerned with the continuing destruction of this planet. An education package which allows discussion on ultraviolet radiation, sunshine, atmospheric pollution, ozone depletion, skin and the inevitable rise in skin cancer may enhance understanding and motivation to modify behaviour. Only then would it make sense to introduce the young to normal moles, malignant melanoma and their main differences.

Preventive strategies can then be discussed which should include the following important points:

- Regular use of High Sun Protection Factor Sunscreen (SPF 15 or more). Tan develops slowly as sunscreens effectively absorb harmful UV rays thus burning is avoided. Waterproof products are also available.
- Use of hats, tee-shirts and parasols. Swimming in tee-shirts is fashionable today and should be encouraged.
- Discourage excessive sun exposure between 11.00 and 15.00 hours (In the UK as well as abroad).
- The importance of protecting at-risk groups: children, fair skinned, persons with family history of melanoma or dysplastic naevus syndrome, persons who have skin which burn easily. Melanoma is twice as common in females as it is in males.

Secondary prevention

The whole ethos of secondary prevention lies in screening for early disease. Examples of secondary prevention programmes are the cervical and breast screening services which are now well established throughout the UK.

To facilitate secondary prevention of disease, contact must be made with those at-risk. Health education programmes, therefore, are an integral part of any secondary preventive strategy as they alert the target population. Such programmes on skin cancer have been commonplace in Australia and USA for more than three decades and have had a profound effect in reducing the mortality rates of melanoma despite increasing incidences. Most of the education is now directed towards children and adolescents eg, *Slip, Slap, Slop* (Australia) and *Teach them sun sense now – avoid skin cancer later* (USA).

Following a recent Cancer Research Campaign initiative an increasing number of screening clinics and public education programmes are being developed specifically for the early recognition and treatment of melanoma. It is anticipated that these health education campaigns will be successful as melanoma is visible on the skin surface. The major warning signs of melanoma: change in size, shape and/or colour may alert individuals, family members, friends, colleagues and health professionals as to the sinister nature of the lesion. Encouragement to seek medical advice quickly can then be offered, while the tumour is at a potentially curable stage. Children and adolescents should be advised to examine the moles on their bodies (and each other). To 'be a mole watcher – for life' is recommended by the Cancer Research Campaign and dermatologists. In learning and realising the normal growth and development of their own moles the recognition of any abnormal change should follow. Table 1 outlines the 7 warning signs of malignant melanoma:

Table 1. Seven warnings of malignant melanoma

1. Growth. Is the new or existing mole growing larger? Ordinary moles gradually mature or grow throughout childhood and adolescence. Normal moles do not usually grow larger in adulthood.

2. Irregular edge. Normal moles have a smooth, regular outline.

3. Colour variation. Normal moles usually only have one or two hues of brown within them.

4. Size. Normal moles usually are of uniform size and less than 0.5cm in diameter. Melanoma is often greater than 1.0cm in diameter.

5. Inflammation. Normal moles do not show any surrounding or underlying inflammation.

6. Bleeding/oozing/crusting. Normal moles do not bleed, ooze or crust spontaneously.

7. Itch. Normal moles are not usually itchy or painful.

Where education has been successful the expected outcomes will be that adolescents and young adults will be able to:
- State the 7 early warning signs of malignant melanoma.
- State the environmental and lifestyle factors which predispose to the disease.
- List the community resources for information about melanoma, its prevention and early detection.
- Describe plans to alter behaviours/lifestyles to decrease risk factors.
- Carry out regular 'mole-checks', and seek medical advice immediately if you recognise any of the early warning signs.

- Be aware of current methods of treatment and expected outcomes. Understand that early surgical treatment can facilitate a cure.

Encouraging mole watching

The implementation of primary and secondary preventive strategies regarding malignant melanoma is rapidly gathering momentum due to increasing incidences worldwide in the white adult population. There is no doubt that the main target groups for any health education are children, adolescents and their parents. Nurses throughout our profession can assist in delivering a health education message by actively encouraging the young to demonstrate a healthy respect for the sun and be molewatchers for life.

References

Breslow, A. (1970) Thickness, cross-sectional area and depth of invasion in the prognosis of cutaneous melanoma. *Ann. Surg.* **172**, 902–8.

Dubin, N., Moseson M. and Pasternick, B.S. (1986) Epidemiology of malignant melanoma: pigmentary traits, ultraviolet radiation and the identification of high risk populations. *Recent Results Cancer Research*, **102**, 58–75.

Green, A. (1984) Sun exposure and risk of melanoma. *Aust. J. Dermatol.* **25**, 99–102.

Hurwitz, S. (1988) The sun and sunscreen protection: recommendations for children. *J. Dermatol. Surg. Oncol.* **14**, 657–60.

Lew, R.A., Sober, A.J., Cook, N. *et al* (1983) Sunburn, sun exposure and melanoma skin cancer. *J. Dermatol. Surg. Oncol.* **9**, 981–6.

MacKie, R.A., (1989) Malignant Melanoma: A Guide To Early Diagnosis. Stiefel. Chapter 2, 6–10.

Muir-Gray, J.A. and Fowler, G. (1984) *Essentials of Preventive Medicine.* Blackwell Scientific, Oxford, Chap. 4, 45–50.

Rhodes, A.R., Weinstock, M.A., Fitzpatrick, T.B. *et al* (1987) Risk factors for cutaneous melanoma: a practical method of recognising predisposed individuals. *J.A.M.A.*, **258**, 3146–54.

White, G. (1977) *Social Processes: Socialisation.* Longman, New York. Chapters 1 and 2, 1–39.

Bibliography

Cancer Research Campaign (1989) *Malignant Melanoma Factsheets* Nos 4.1 and 4.2

Cancer Research Campaign (1986) A Co-ordinated Programme to Evaluate the Role of Education in Early Detection of Malignant Melanoma. (Unpublished Literature).

Chanda J. (1986) The Clinical Recognition and Prognostic Factors of Primary Cutaneous Malignant Melanoma. *Medical Clinics of N. America.* **70**, 1.

Imperial Cancer Research Fund (1990) *Sun Cool:Sun, Skin, Moles and Melanoma.* Education Literature. I.C.R.F., London.

Magnus, K. (1987) Epidemiology of malignant melanoma of the skin. In *Cutaneous Melanoma: Status of Knowledge and Future Perspectives.* (Eds) Veronesi, Cascinelli & Santinami. Part 1, 1–13.

Wessex Cancer Trust (1990) *Monty Mole's Marvellous Mission.* Colour and Learn Booklet. Wessex Cancer Trust, Southampton.

25
What is diabetes?

Sheila Reading, MSc, BSc (Hons), RGN, PGCEA
Nurse Teacher, Southampton University College of Nursing and Midwifery

Causes and classification

The cause, or causes, of diabetes are not completely understood, although genetic, environmental and immunological factors are thought to be involved. For a more detailed discussion refer to 'Caring for the Patient with Diabetes', Chapter 1 (Kinson and Nattrass, 1984).

In the past the classification of diabetes has led to much confusion. Terms such as 'severe', 'moderate' or 'mild' diabetes depending on presenting symptoms, and 'juvenile onset' or 'maturity onset' diabetes depending on the person's age at presentation, are misleading and ambiguous. For example, juvenile onset diabetes, usually inferring insulin dependent diabetes (IDD), can develop at any age. The present classification put forward by the National Diabetes Data Group (1979) and accepted by the WHO (1980) is based on our present knowledge of aetiology, but still contains a few anomalies and can only be used where the relevant investigations have been carried out. Diabetes is classified primarily according to clinical descriptions, but the terms Type 1 and Type 2 diabetes indicate the underlying aetiology are also included, Type 1 usually being associated with IDD and Type 2 with NIDD. (Keen, 1983).

Insulin dependent diabetes (IDD)   Characterised by an insulin insufficiency caused by a lack of functional beta cells in the pancreas and requiring insulin injections for survival.

Non insulin dependent diabetes (NIDD)   Characterised by a relative insulin deficiency often related to a defective beta cell secretory response (Montague, 1983). Dietary control, or dietary control plus oral hypoglycaemic drugs, will achieve normal blood glucose levels.

About 25 per cent of people with diabetes are insulin dependent. Non insulin dependent diabetes is often considered to be a milder form of diabetes, but retinal, neurological and renal complications are just as likely to occur. For a summary of the two types see Table 1.

The role of insulin

Insulin is a hormone secreted by the ß (beta) cells of the islets of Langerhans in the pancreas. It is of central importance in carbohydrate metabolism and normally maintains blood glucose concentrations within the range of 2.6 to 6.6 mmols/litre. Insulin secretion is closely linked with

Type of Diabetes	Insulin Dependent Diabetes	Non Insulin Dependent Diabetes
Insulin Deficiency	Absolute.	Relative.
Treatment	Diet and insulin injections.	Diet alone or diet and oral hypoglycaemic agents.
Clinical Onset	Rapid/severe symptoms of thirst polyuria, weight loss and fatigue. Ketones present in urine.	Slow, insidious onset can precede diagnosis by months. Symptoms mild or non-existent. Ketones not present in urine.
Age at diagnosis	Usually, but not invariably the patient is under 30 years of age.	Usually, but not invariably the patient is over 40 years of age.
Weight	Tend to be thin.	Tend to be overweight.

Table 1. Differences between the two types of diabetes.

food intake. Following a meal, when nutrients are absorbed into the blood stream, the circulating levels of insulin rise. Glucose levels are maintained below 6.6mmols/litre by insulin inhibiting glucose production from the liver and stimulating glucose utilisation and storage.

As the levels of circulating insulin decrease in response to reduced nutrients in the blood stream, the situation is reversed to maintain the blood glucose level above 2.6mmols/litre.

Insulin also has a role in protein and fat metabolism. Protein synthesis and fat synthesis and storage are stimulated by the action of insulin and the breakdown of both are inhibited by insulin (Figure 1).

Results of insulin deficiency

When insulin is deficient, blood glucose levels rise. When the blood glucose level exceeds the renal threshold (about 10mmols/litre) glucose appears in the urine and causes an osmotic diuresis leading to polyuria and thirst. In severe insulin deficiency fat is broken down to supply energy and ketones are produced leading to rapid breathing, nausea, and vomiting. The end results are coma and death. The extreme picture usually occurs among true IDD patients; paradoxically NIDD patients may remain asymptomatic despite a damaging level of blood glucose.

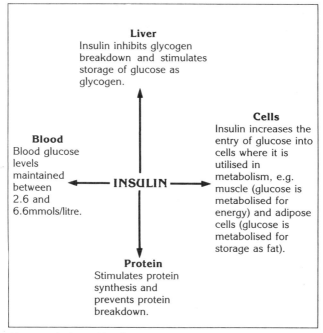

Figure 1. Actions of insulin.

Symptoms of diabetes

Polyuria — excess water is lost as glucose is excreted in the urine.

Polydipsia and dehydration — due to excess water depletion caused by osmotic diuresis.

Nausea and vomiting — the exact cause is unkown but is probably due to the disturbed metabolism of carbohydrates, protein and fat, resulting in abnormal levels of glucose, ketone bodies and amino acids in the blood.

Tiredness — glucose is not being metabolised for energy.

Pruritis vulvae, balanitis and/or urinary tract infection — glucose in the urine increases the possibility of infection (usually yeast infections).

Muscle weakness and loss of weight — due to breakdown of protein and fat; only in cases of absolute insulin deficiency.

Formation of ketone bodies progressing to keto-acidosis/coma/death — only in cases of absolute insulin deficiency.

Diagnosis

Although symptoms vary depending on the type, there always exists a raised blood glucose concentration. Normally a random blood glucose greater than 11mmols/litre in the presence of symptoms establishes a diagnosis of diabetes. A fasting blood glucose level above 8mmols/litre is also diagnostic (WHO criteria). In a few cases the fasting blood glucose result may be equivocal, particularly if symptoms are not present, and an oral glucose tolerance test may be necessary to establish a diagnosis.

Treatment and management

The aims of treatment and management are relief of symptoms and prevention of long term complications, which are achieved by good control of blood glucose; education of the patient to enable effective self care and regular surveillance to monitor blood glucose and detect and treat complications which may occur.

It is essential that everyone with diabetes is educated to understand their condition and the principles of diet and treatment. There is a lot to learn, but unless patients are fully involved in their own care, the aims of treatment are unlikely to be achieved. A means of assessing the success of management should always be available to the patient in his home so that adjustments can be made to diet, or if applicable the insulin dose, to achieve normal blood glucose levels.

Insulin dependent diabetes   Treatment consists of insulin injections and diet to control of blood glucose and relief of symptoms. The aim is to achieve normal blood glucose levels by balancing food intake, insulin dose and timing, and exercise.

Non insulin dependent diabetes   Often obesity is the problem and the first line of action is to advise a sugar free low calorie diet, which may control blood glucose levels. Hypoglycaemic agents (sulphonylureas or biguanides) should only be prescribed if the patient cannot achieve blood glucose control despite weight loss, or if symptoms continue.

Dietary Principles   Carbohydrate restriction used to be the accepted means of dietary advice but *is no longer advocated*. This is because low carbohydrate diets tend to be supplemented by diets high in fat to achieve an adequate calorie intake and this policy may be bad for the cardiovascular system. Instead, decreased fat intake and increased carbohydrate from foodstuffs rich in fibre such as wholemeal bread and pastas, legumes and pulses is encouraged. A high fibre diet slows down the rate of digestion and therefore the rate of absorption of glucose into the blood. The dietitian should advise each person individually, and recommend how much carbohydrate should be eaten, depending on lifestyle and calorie requirements. Those requiring insulin should take equivalent amounts of carbohydrate at roughly the same time each day to balance the insulin regime, taking account of physical activity patterns.

References

Keen, H. (1983) Criteria and classification of diabetes mellitus. In: Mann, J.I., Pyorala, K. and Teucher, A. (Eds) *Diabetes in Epidemiological Perspective*. Churchill Livingstone, Edinburgh.

Kinson, J. and Nattrass, M. (1984) *Caring for the Diabetic Patient*. Churchill Livingstone, Edinburgh.

Montague, W. (1983) *Diabetes and the Endocrine Pancreas. A biochemical approach*. Croom Helm, London.

National Diabetes Data Group (1979) Classification and diagnosis of diabetes mellitus and other categories of glucose intolerance. *Diabetes*, **28**, 1039.

World Health Organisation Expert Committee on Diabetes Mellitus (1980) Second Report, WHO, Technical Report Series, No. 646.

Bibliography

Mann, J. (1982) *The Diabetics Diet Book*. Martin Dunitz, London.
A useful guide emphasising the use of high fibre foods.

26

An extra source of conflict? Diabetes in adolescence

Julie Smith, BSc, RGN, RHV

Previously Diabetes Specialist Nurse, Peterborough Health Authority and currently undertaking a Postgraduate Certificate in Education, Nottingham University

Diabetes is a lifelong condition requiring daily treatment which is not part of an accepted 'normal' lifestyle. For an adolescent, this entails daily insulin injections, regular blood glucose monitoring and awareness of hyperglycaemia and hypoglycaemia. Diabetics also have to plan ahead, taking adequate precautions for exercise, travel, pregnancy and contraception and can face restrictions on driving, employment and financial arrangements. This has serious implications for adolescent diabetics who face added responsibility when they are experiencing independence for the first time.

Diabetes causes some inconvenience to all sufferers, but especially for adolescents, who are in a transition period often viewed as traumatic. Adolescence is a period of rapid physical and psychological development. The physical development is largely centred around hormonal actions and the attainment of puberty, before which long-term complications of diabetes are rare. Loss of control can appear at puberty, particularly in young women in whom ketoacidosis appears to be more common. Although long-term complications are rare before puberty, poor control can lead to poor physical development, especially in terms of growth.

The psychological development in adolescence marks the change from being a child to becoming an adult – a move from a dependent to an independent state. Diabetes causes extra difficulty because the individual is forced to rely on management of their condition to stay alive. The contradiction between the desired independent state and an enforced dependent state can lead to resentment, rebellion and anger. This can cause a changing relationship with parents, usually seen as a 'difficult' stage, and the priorities of parents and adolescents may differ. Parents, for example, may view attendance at a diabetic clinic as important, while most adolescents are more concerned with fashion and making friends of the opposite sex. This is a normal part of the socialisation process, and peer group pressure and approval is of the utmost importance in terms of fashion and lifestyle, all of which diabetes can interfere with. Shoes that are likely to be beneficial in preventing foot problems are not necessarily fashionable! Even legislation allowing an individual to have sexual intercourse or to buy alcohol have implications for the management of diabetes.

The conflicting demands between dependence and independence can lead to stress. Adolescents are particularly vulnerable as they are beginning to form their own identity and need careful treatment if this is to be accomplished successfully. Various aspects of the management of diabetes can be problematic to adolescents, but there are practical ways in which nurses may help.

Insulin therapy

For adolescents, insulin injections can be time-consuming, inconvenient and embarrassing. It is not unusual for insulin injections to be omitted over a period of time for these very reasons.

All diabetics are entitled to free insulin syringes on prescription, and plastic disposable syringes are simple to use and require no sterilisation, so they are less trouble to administer. Devices are also available on prescription for cutting off and retaining the needle away from the barrel of the syringe, preventing both reuse and the spread of infection. Pen devices are available for administering insulin, which is stored in an attached cartridge. They are easy to carry and do not require filling for each injection. Devices containing fast-acting insulin require three to four injections daily plus an additional injection of longer-acting insulin to provide background cover. This approach allows for greater flexibility and adaptation to a chosen lifestyle. A recent trial by Jenkins *et al* (1989) showed an improvement in both metabolic control and acceptability when one such device was used by adolescents.

Adolescents need encouragement from qualified professionals such as nurse specialists or doctors to help them adjust the dose safely as required for the varying demands of illness, eating out and exercise. Experimentation with dosage enables them to learn how to cope independently. In the non-diabetic, insulin secretion varies with different activities depending upon the blood glucose level, and the same principles may be applied to the diabetic: guidelines on insulin adjustment are available from their own doctor (GP or hospital consultant) and the insulin manufacturers. Many health authorities have diabetic care teams consisting of a diabetologist, diabetic specialist nurses and dietitians who are all available to give advice on any aspect of management. Burton (1988) provides a useful account of insulin preparations available.

Encouragement should be given to vary the sites of injection: suitable areas are the arms, abdomen, buttocks, thighs and calfs, otherwise the insulin will not be properly absorbed; the area will become hard and unsightly lumps develop – a potential problem for the fashion conscious teenager. Swabbing the injection site prior to giving the insulin subcutaneously at a 90 degree angle also hardens the skin and should be discouraged.

A few adolescents develop an aversion to injecting because they find it painful. This is often due to incorrect injection technique, and reinforcement of the correct technique is usually enough to overcome it. True needle phobia is rare, but there are commercially produced aids to injecting which have been successfully used by some individuals.

Blood glucose monitoring

Adolescents need reliable information about their blood glucose levels if they are to safely adjust their insulin dosage. This is particularly important if they are going through a period of rapid growth or have an acute illness, both of which require increased insulin. Many adolescents find that blood testing is more inconvenient and painful than insulin injections, and a compromise may have to be reached. Blood testing strips and most needles for finger-pricking are now available on prescription, and mechanical devices for finger-pricking and electronic meters are available commercially. The side of the little and ring fingers are the least painful to prick and a delay of a few seconds should be allowed before milking the finger to form a large drop. This often prevents the finger being pricked twice! The manufacturer's instructions should be followed carefully with regard to the timing and materials required, and results must be accurately recorded and tests taken at different times of the day. The importance of blood tests to the individual, rather than the doctor, should be stressed, and encouragement given for *honest* recording of results – a few honest results are infinitely more valuable than a page of neatly recorded false ones! Gadgets and electronic meters may provide an impetus for some youngsters to blood test, but they need to be properly cleaned and calibrated and the manufacturer's instructions carefully followed. If blood glucose testing still proves unacceptable, then urine testing may have to be considered. This method is not as reliable because of differing renal thresholds, the time delay between the urine being produced and tested and a less accurate recording scale.

It is only by testing that an accurate assessment of the diabetic condition can be made. Blood glucose testing, for example, will give an immediate quantifiable result in the case of suspected hypoglycaemia. An HbAI (glycosylated haemoglobin) will give an estimation of glycaemic control for the previous few weeks and a sample of venous blood may be obtained at clinic visits.

Hypoglycaemia

Many adolescents find hypoglycaemic attacks uncomfortable and embarrassing. The main causes are too much injected insulin, deficiency of carbohydrate or too much physical excerise. Symptoms vary from person to person, but consist primarily of shaking, sweating, pallor, palpitations, hunger, tingling around the mouth, changes in behaviour and vagueness. Many of these symptoms are due to a surge of adrenalin as the body tries to compensate for the lack of glucose by secreting growth hormones, steroids, adrenalin and glucagon. All adolescents should be encouraged to carry glucose in the form of tablets and to wear some form of identification, even though this will mark them out as different from their friends. Hypoglycaemia is treated by first relieving the symptoms with a fast-acting carbohydrate (eg, glucose), followed by a longer acting form such as a wholemeal sandwich. In severe attacks hypoglycaemia can cause unconsciousness and intramuscular glucagon should be administered and oral medicine avoided. The glucagon may take several minutes to act, and nausea and vomiting may occur, but unlike intravenous dextrose, there is no potential damage to the vein using glucagon. Reassurance may be given that death from hypoglycaemia is rare and even if treatment is not given, recovery does follow but may take several hours. Exceptions are due to underlying liver disease or following the ingestion of large quantities of alcohol. Alcohol causes a drop in blood glucose levels (although many alcoholic drinks are a combination of both sugar and alcohol) and hinders the liver's ability to produce glucose. Its action may be delayed by several hours, and the symptoms of hypoglycaemia and being drunk are difficult to distinguish. Regular blood glucose monitoring may indicate a pattern of hypoglycaemia, so steps can be taken to prevent its occurrence.

Ketoacidosis

Hyperglycaemia can lead to the life-threatening condition of ketoacidosis. This is most likely to occur during periods of acute illness or if insulin injections are omitted over a period of time – a possible sign of adolescent rebellion. Ketoacidosis results when the body is unable to utilise glucose as an energy source due to lack of insulin, and fat is used as an energy supply. Incomplete metabolism of fat leads to production of ketones which, if they build up, are toxic and may lead to coma and death. Signs of ketoacidosis are polyuria, polydipsia, vomiting, abdominal pain and deep sighing (Kussmaul's) respirations. Hospital admission is necessary, and treatment consists of rehydration, insulin therapy and balance of electrolytes. If an adolescent has raised blood glucose and is acutely ill, he or she should be advised to increase the frequency of blood glucose monitoring, replace carbohydrate intake with sweetened fluids and *never* to stop insulin – it is likely an increase will be necessary. Testing strips are available to detect the presence of ketones in the urine, and all adolescents should be given a packet for use in emergencies. Ketones also have a characteristic smell resembling pear-drops and can be smelt on the breath. Medical advice should be sought if they are present.

Living with diabetes

Diet   The same dietary recommendations apply to adolescents with diabetes as to everyone else: high complex carbohydrate, fibre and low fat, but dietary advice is individual to the person and there can be no set regime. Some dietitians advocate the use of carbohydrate exchanges and others do not, so nurses giving dietary advice to adolescents may be advised to liaise with the dietitian concerned, to ensure they do not give conflicting advice (Kinmouth *et al*, 1989)

Many adolescents 'cheat' in their diets (as do many adults) but provided this happens infrequently, it is unlikely to cause any real harm. Recent guidelines suggest a small amount of added sucrose in the diet is unlikely to cause major detriment (Jenkins *et al*, 1989), but a wide range of artificial sweeteners is also available. Diabetic products, however, are not encouraged as they may cause weight gain, help develop a sweet tooth and can contain sorbitol which causes gastrointestinal disturbances in susceptible individuals. Alcohol is allowed in moderation, but should never be substituted for carbohydrate allowance or taken on an empty stomach, because of the risk of hypoglycaemia. Diabetic lager, low alcohol products (which have a high simple carbohydrate content), sweet wines, sherries and liqueurs are also not recommended. Adolescents often enjoy fast foods and fizzy drinks, so a carbohydrate/calories check list relating to these is available from the British Diabetic Association (BDA).

Eating out and socialising are important to many adolescents, and insulins should be adjusted to allow for this. A diabetic on twice daily injections who is planning a late evening meal out should eat a snack at the time they would normally take their evening insulin, which should then be taken 30 minutes before the meal. If a social event includes dancing, it is advisable to slightly increase the amount of carbohydrate taken.

Threatening adolescents with development of complications if they do not improve their control is unlikely to achieve any positive effects; it is more likely to drive them away. Regular attendance at clinic sessions for screening is an important way of making contact. Sessions need not resemble traditional adult diabetic clinics: up-to-date topical magazines and background chart music can be provided, and adolescents can be encouraged to attend unaccompanied by their parents. The emphasis should also be on health rather than disease.

Exercise and sport   Young people with diabetes should be encouraged to exercise, although there is a risk of hypoglycaemia in the adequately-insulinised (a rise in blood glucose can result in people who are under-insulinised). Hypoglycaemia can occur during or after exercise, and it is necessary to either increase carbohydrate and/or reduce insulin. The type of carbohydrate will depend upon the type of exercise undertaken: fast-acting for vigorous, short-lived activity such as squash and slower-acting carbohydrate for more prolonged exercise. It may be necessary to take a combination of the two, and glucose should always be available in the form of tablets or drink.

Travel/holidays   Travel and holidays abroad are part of many adolescents' lives and a few precautions are necessary for those with diabetes. Identification in the form of a card or jewellery may prevent embarrassment at customs if needles and syringes are being carried and it is wise to take more than enough supplies for the whole holiday, even though insulin is available internationally. On aeroplanes, insulin should be carried in the hand luggage to avoid it arriving in Acapulco when the diabetic is in Athens! Also, the temperatures in aircraft holds can cause insulin to freeze.

It may be necessary to alter insulin dosage if travel crosses time zones; the diabetic team will be able to advise on this. In the case of travel sickness or stomach upsets abroad, the same advice as for hyperglycaemia applies. Blood glucose monitoring is important on holiday, as the change in temperatures may mean insulin doses need to be changed, so it should be emphasised that holidays do not mean a rest from diabetes too.

The BDA organise activity holidays for young diabetics with the aim of providing a good holiday and promoting education and independence. They are staffed by doctors, nurses and dietitians, and also provide useful learning experiences for professionals. The Youth Diabetes Project provides outdoor activity courses at Firbush, Scotland for 16-25 year-olds, holds an annual conference and encourages self-help groups. A medical workshop is also held at Firbush.

Driving   Diabetics must notify the DVLC of their condition and the driving licence is renewed every three years after checking for severe hypoglycaemia with their doctor. Licences may not be held for heavy goods vehicles, passenger service vehicles and piloting. If hypoglycaemia occurs while driving, it is essential to turn off the engine and get out of the car where it is safe to do so.

School   The BDA produce a school pack providing information to teachers. Commonly held worries relate to hypoglycaemia and diet.

Employment   A recent survey by Robinson (1989) has shown that 16-25 year-olds with diabetes are more likely to be or have been unemployed, even though they are less likely to take time off sick than non-diabetics. Some employers discriminate against diabetics, which makes some young people unwilling to declare their condition, which, of course, can lead to problems in itself. It is possible for people with diabetes to register as disabled, and some firms take a designated number of disabled employees. Certain occupations exclude those with diabetes, including the police and armed services, while shift work may require adjustment to dietary and insulin patterns.

Finance   Diabetes can have implications for insurance (eg, life, travel, motor and mortages) so it is well worth shopping around. All diabetics are exempt from prescription charges and, in cases of hardship, travel expenses to hospital appointments may be refundable.

Contraception and pregnancy   Poorly controlled diabetes during pregnancy is associated with babies of large birthweight and a higher rate of congenital malformations and stillbirth due to hyperglycaemia. Ideally, excellent control should be attained prior to conception and certainly maintained during pregnancy. Insulin requirements may decrease during the first trimester and then increase until the end of the pregnancy. After birth, these will return to the pre-pregnancy requirements for good control. Breast feeding is encouraged and extra carbohydrate will be necessary. A pregnancy pack is available from the BDA.

Most forms of contraception can be used, although some doctors do not advocate the use of the intrauterine device (coil) or oral contraception high in oestrogen: the progesterone only or 'mini-pill' is preferred. Some young women find their blood glucose level fluctuates with menstruation and they need to adjust their insulin accordingly.

A realistic approach

Adolescence is a difficult time for anyone, but for those with diabetes to manage, it can become fraught unless good support is available. At such vulnerable times, adolescents may turn to nurses for help. It is important that this is not given in an authoritarian, restrictive way – this will do nothing for the relationship, whereas being realistic might. Positive reinforcement and praise, listening and treating young people as adults are all important and will encourage them to stay in contact even if there is a short-term loss of control. Education need not be boring: experiential learning can take the form of meals out and other group activities. Even if manipulation and experimentation does occur (with 'cheating', false blood glucose results, non-attendance at clinics and omitting injections), this can still be perceived as a learning experience, although safety is of the utmost importance.

Many areas have diabetic healthcare teams – doctors, diabetes specialist nurses (working in both hospital and the community), dietitians, chiropodists and sometimes psychologists, all of whom are available as a resource to help nurses give adolescents the support they need in this transitional period of their lives.

References

Burton, S. (1988) Drug update: the insulins. *The Professional Nurse*, **3**, 9, 335–38.
Davies, R. *et al* (1989) Progress in the youth diabetes project. *Practical Diabetes*, **6**, 6, 262–63.
Jenkins, H. *et al* (1989) A study of metabolic control and patient acceptability in adolescent diabetics using the Novopen. *Practical Diabetes*, **6**, 1, 14–15.
Kinmouth, A.L. *et al* (1989) Dietary recommendations for children and adolescents with diabetes. *Diabetes*, **6**, 6, 537–47.
Robinson, N. (1989) *Birth to Old Age – Health in Transition*. OUP, Milton Keynes.

Robinson, N. (1989) Working for diabetes. *Balance*, Oct/Nov, 28–31.
U 205 (1985) *Birth to Old Age – Health in Transition*. OUP, Milton Keynes.

Bibliography
Day, D.L., (1986) Insulin Dependent Diabetes. Thorsons Publishing Group, Wellingborough and BDA, London.
Primarily written for patients, but useful for healthcare professionals.
Kinson, J. and Nattrass, M. (1984) Caring for the Diabetic Patient. Churchill Livingstone, Edinburgh.
This book is written specifically for nurses and links theory to practice.
Sonksen, P., Fox, C. and Judd, S. (1985) The Diabetes Reference Book. Harper and Row, London.
Question and answer format.
Tattersall, R. (1986) Diabetes. Churchill Livingstone, Edinburgh.
A good practical guide.
Balance. Bimonthly magazine of the BDA.
Contains up-to-date practical information and carries details of new products and research. Available from newsagents or by joining the BDA.
Practical Diabetes, published by the Newbourne Group. Focuses on the multidisciplinary healthcare team. Free circulation to interested professionals.

Useful addresses
British Diabetic Association, 10 Queen Anne Street, London W1M 0BD. Te: 071-323 1531.
Provides advice and information about all aspects of diabetes, and has a youth department and education section for professionals.
English National Board for Nursing, Midwifery and Health Visiting, Victory House, 170 Tottenham Court Road, London W1T 0HA. Tel. 071-388 3131.
Advice about ENB course 928 – a short course on diabetic nursing.
RCN Association of Nursing Practice, Royal College of Nursing, 20 Cavendish Square, London W1M 0AB. Tel. 071-409 3333.
Diabetes nursing forum – annual conferences and newsletters.

27

Breast cancer screening: women's reluctance to attend

Patricia A. Black, BA (Hons), RGN
Health Visitor Student (Dip HV), South Bank Polytechnic

Mass screening of the population at risk (Table 1) undoubtedly improves survival chances for breast cancer sufferers by detecting early tumours, as Adami's study in Sweden (1986) indicates. But any screening programme is only as effective as the number of people who participate in it. A study of individuals who accept or reject screening procedures showed that women were more likely to attend if personally invited, but even if invited only 57.3 per cent did so (Hobbs et al, 1980).

Fear is one possible reason for low participation, but fear of what? Of cancer itself or of the mutilating surgery that may be carried out to cure it? In western culture, the breast has special sexual significance and its removal has a tremendous psychological effect, exceeding the 'normal' period of mourning which follows loss of a body part (Rosen, 1950).

- Early menarche.
- Late age at first pregnancy.
- Nulliparity.
- Upper social class.
- Previous history of benign breast disease.
- Family history of breast cancer.
- Abnormality in steroid metabolism resulting in outputs of C 19 urinary steroids.

Table 1. Women at risk.

Screening programme

A screening programme must press home the fact that cancer is curable if detected at an early stage. It must include information on new techniques and be aimed at the general population and health professionals.

In saying that most breast lumps are not malignant, health care professionals must be aware that there are two ways a person may react. If a woman finds a lump in her breast she may be encouraged to attend a clinic to have it investigated as the chances are that it is benign; but on the other hand she may reason that if the chances are that it is benign then why bother to attend clinic in the first place?

Lumpectomy, with or without radiotherapy, is a viable alternative in many instances, but women are often justifiably afraid that breast amputation will be the only alternative offered. Some may consider this to be at least as bad as the disease itself. According to Gazet et al (1985) almost three-quarters of British surgeons still opt for mastectomy as the treatment of choice for 75-100 per cent of their patients, as it gives a low rate of recurrence. However, as Harris (1984) and Pickren (1984) point out, breast conservation has a similarly favourable prognosis.

Most breast conservation techniques are carried out in major breast cancer treatment centres. It seems probable that lack of knowledge about new techniques on the part of health care professionals outside these centres is one reason for this; with lack of specialist radiotherapy equipment being another. If health care professionals and women at risk become aware of treatment alternatives they can create a 'demand' for equipment. Health authorities may be reluctant to invest in expensive equipment, but it can be proved cost effective in the long term.

Women might be motivated to attend clinics and overcome fear of disfigurement if services other than breast screening were offered. The concept of 'Well Woman Clinics' could be enlarged to include cervical and coronary heart disease screening as well as counsellors to assist women to come to terms with unfavourable test results.

Information about alternative treatments for early detected breast cancers could be provided, reducing the perceived inevitability of mutilating surgery. More women may then be persuaded to attend clinics.

Morris (1979) has shown that the incidence of psychological morbidity is higher if a woman is not allowed time to adjust to breast loss. To minimise the possibility of psychological disturbance when mastectomy is unavoidable, counselling throughout all stages from diagnosis onwards for both the woman and her partner is crucial. Further, the practice of carrying out mastectomy immediately after a positive 'frozen section' biopsy should be abolished unless exceptional medical circumstances dictate otherwise, as this does not allow the vital adjustment period.

References

Adami, H.O. *et al* (1986) Temporal trends in breast cancer survival in Sweden: significant improvement in 20 years. *JNCI*, **76**, 653–9.

Gazet, J.C., Rainsbury, R.M., Ford, H.T., Powles, T.J. and Coombes, R.C. (1985) Survey of treatment of primary breast cancer in Great Britain. *British Medical Journal*, **290**, 6484, 1793–5.

Harris, J.R. *et al* (1984) Time, course and prognosis of local recurrence following primary radiation therapy for early breast cancer. *Journal Clin. Oncol.* **2**, 1, 37–41.

Hobbs, P. *et al* (1980) Acceptors and rejectors of an invitation to undergo breast screening compared with those who referred themselves. *Journal of Epidemiology and Community Health*, **34**, 19–22.

Morris, T. (1979) Psychological adjustment to mastectomy. *Cancer Treatment Reviews*, **6**, 41–61.

Pickren, J.W. (1984) Lumpectomy for mammary carcinoma: a retrospective analysis of 40 presumptive candidates from a surgical series. *Cancer*, **15**, 54, 8, 1692–5.

Rosen, V.H. (1950) The role of denial in acute postoperative affective reactions following removal of body parts. *Psychosom. Med.*, **12**, 356.

Handout: a guide to examining your breasts

If you find a lump or anything unusual in your breast, it isn't likely to be serious.

But if it is, the earlier you find it, the easier the cure.

The treatment options now available if it is breast cancer are:

- lumpectomy;
- mastectomy;
- chemotherapy;
- radiotherapy.

Sometimes a combination of these is used. Chemotherapy – the use of drugs to attack the cancer – is not usually used for periods of more than six months.

Mastectomy is more likely to be necessary if the lump is large, which is why screening is so important. Small lumps may only need lumpectomy – removal of just the lump and surrounding tissue – with or without radiotherapy, or possibly only chemotherapy, so the sooner they are detected the more likely you are to keep your breast.

Reconstruction

If a mastectomy is suggested, you may want to discuss the possibility of breast reconstruction. This uses grafts of skin and muscle with the insertion of a silicon implant to rebuild the breast.

It is in your interest to examine your breasts monthly as shown in this handout, especially if you are in an increased risk category.

Increased risk categories

1. Family history of breast cancer.
2. Childlessness.
3. First pregnancy at 35+.
4. Periods beginning before age 12 years.

It's important

It takes very little time each month to check for yourself that your breasts are healthy. It's a simple and easy routine and it's important to make it a habit.

By examining your breasts regularly, you get to know what is normal for you. They you'll find it easy to spot any changes.

If you do find something wrong, you'll be able to get treatment early. In most cases it won't be cancer but just a cyst or growth which can be dealt with very easily especially when it's found early. If it is cancer, then early treatment gives you the best chance of a complete cure.

When to examine your breasts

The best time to examine your breasts is just after a period, when your breasts are usually softest and no longer tender. Or, if you've stopped having periods, choose a day in the month you'll be able to remember, like the first day or the last. The important thing is to examine your breasts regularly, at the same time each month.

There are two stages to examining your breasts. The first is looking and the second is feeling.

Looking

When you examine your breasts you're looking for anything that's unusual. For this, looking is just as important as feeling.

Undress to the waist and sit or stand in front of a mirror in a good light. When you look at your breasts, remember that no two are the same – not even your own two. One will probably be slightly larger than the other, and one a little lower on the chest.

Here's what to look for:

- any change in the size of either breast;

- any change in either nipple;

- bleeding or discharge from either nipple;

- any unusual dimple or puckering on the breast or nipple;

- veins standing out more than is usual for you.

Examining your breasts
Remember

- If you do find a lump, it is most likely to be harmless.

- If it is cancerous, the quicker it is diagnosed, the more likely you are to keep your breast.

1. First let your arms hang loosely by your sides and look at your breasts in the mirror.

2. Next raise your arms above your head. Watch in the mirror as you turn from side to side to see your breasts from different angles.

3. Now look down at your breasts and squeeze each nipple gently to check for any bleeding or discharge that's unusual for you.

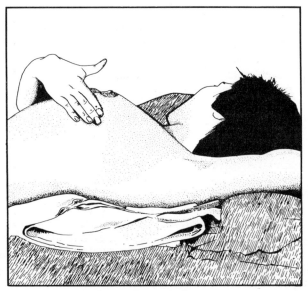

4. Lie down on your bed and make yourself comfortable with your head on a pillow. Examine one breast at a time.

    Put a folded towel under your shoulder-blade on the side you are examining. This helps to spread the breast tissue so that it is easier to examine. Use your right hand to examine your left breast and vice versa. Put the hand you're not using under year head.

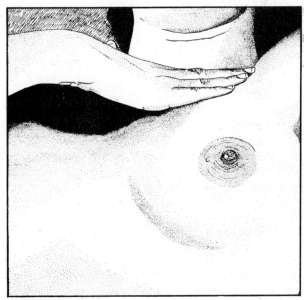

5. Keep your fingers together and use the flat of the fingers, not the tips. Start from the collarbone above your breast.

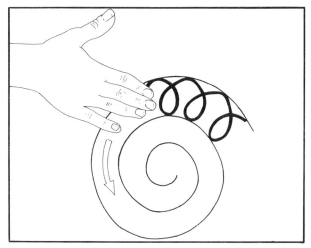

6. Trace a continuous spiral round your breast moving your fingers in small circles. Feel gently but firmly for any unusual lump or thickening.

   Work right round the outside of your breast first. When you get back to your starting point, work round again in a slightly smaller circle, and so on. Keep on doing this until you have worked right up to the nipple. Make sure you cover every part of your breast.

   You may find a ridge of firm tissue in a half-moon shape under your breast. This is quite normal. It is tissue that develops to help support your breast.

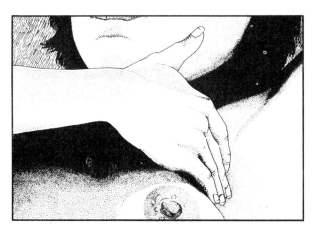

7. Finally, examine your armpit. Still use the flat of your fingers and the same small circular movements to feel for any lumps. Start right up in the hollow or your armpit and gradually work your way down towards your breast. It's important not to forget this last part of the examination.

Any problems?

If you think you've found something unusual in one breast but you're not sure, check the same part of the other breast. If both breasts feel the same, it's probably just the way your breasts are made.

If you still think something may be wrong, then see your doctor. It doesn't matter how uncertain you are. It's far better to see your doctor and set your mind at rest than risk neglecting something serious.

Make a note of where the lump or change is. Arrange to see your doctor within the next few days. In the meantime, try not to keep feeling the lump to see if it has gone away or got any bigger. It's best to leave it alone.

Adapted from A Guide to Examining Your Breasts, with kind permission of the Health Education Authority.

If you would like advice about examining your breasts, ask your doctor, or the nurse or health visitor at your local clinic.

28

Teaching testicular self-examination

Bettina Schäufele, RGN
Currently working as an agency nurse in London, while studying courses in family planning and holistic medicine

Testicular cancer is a relatively rare disease, representing only about one per cent of all cancers diagnosed in men. However, it is the leading cause of death from cancer in males between the age of 15 to 35 years (Blesch, 1986; Carlin, 1986).

In the early stage of the disease the man might notice a painless enlargement of the testicle, complain of a vague 'heaviness' and he might feel a hard, small lump on palpation. Pain is only present at the later stage, when nerves have been infiltrated as the cancer has metastasised to the lymph nodes or bones. The absence of pain initially, combined with a lack of knowledge, often causes men to delay in seeking medical advice (see Table 1).

Provided the cancer is detected and treated at an early stage, the cure rate is up to 100 per cent, which represents one of the success stories of today's oncology (Davies, 1981). Abnormalities of the testicle can be detected effectively by a regular palpation of the scrotum, yet only a small proportion of the male population have heard of testicular self-examination (TSE) and even fewer practise it regularly. A study conducted in Ireland in 1986 involving 500 men of high socioeconomic and educational status showed that 93 per cent of them were unaware that testicular cancer is a common malignancy between the ages of 15 and 40; testicular self-examination was unknown to 92 per cent of the men. Yet 90 per cent of the men said that they would be interested in more information about cancer of the testis and self-examination (Thornhill et al, 1986). The outcome of the study suggests that either the health care team has not assessed men's health education needs and is not providing adequate information, or that the health education message is not reaching the male population.

Cryptorchidism (undescended testicles). Family history of testicular cancer. Previous history of testicular cancer. Caucasian race. Possibly trauma.

Table 1. Increased risk factors for testicular cancer.

The nurse's role

As testicular cancer occurs mainly in young men in the prime of their professional life and probably with young, dependent families, the effects of this disease can have an enormous economic, social and emotional impact. How can nurses increase public awareness of testicular cancer and promote regular self-examination? First, as members of the health care profession, nurses need to look at their own attitudes towards health education. They have to accept their responsibility as health educators and need to maintain an up-to-date knowledge (as laid down in the code of professional conduct by the UKCC). Nurses should also regularly assess and evaluate the effectiveness of their communication skills and be aware of the barriers which possible sexual embarrassment may cause.

We also need to look at men and their position in society. According to Forrester (1986), the traditional male sex stereotype is healthy, strong, independent and dominating. This hidden expectation can set barriers for men in seeking information about health education or preventive health care. It can also prevent them from obtaining prompt medical advice for anything abnormal they might have detected, especially in areas affecting their sexuality. More health authorities should therefore be encouraged to set up 'Well Man' clinics, where men can obtain expert advice and receive regular check-ups. Men are also restricted in the time they can attend such services by their professional lives, and this should be taken into account by arranging evening or Saturday opening hours for such centres.

Finally, nurses must assess how the health education message could be spread among young and mostly healthy men, who rarely come into contact with their local hospital or consult their GP. On school entry, boys should be checked for undescended testicles and their parents need to be made aware of the associated risks. While in secondary school, boys could be introduced to TSE in sex education classes. This knowledge could later on be reinforced in colleges and universities during health care lectures or by promoting preventive medicine with the introductioh of a 'self-care day'. Information boards with regularly changing topics on health and wellbeing could also be set up in the main meeting areas.

Spread the message

Male genitalia are particularly at risk of injury during sport exercises. PE teachers or sports trainers could therefore include information about TSE into their classes (Conklin et al, 1978).

During health screening in factories and companies, occupational nurses could assess the men's knowledge about testicular cancer and could encourage self-examination. Leaflets with detailed information should be available to bridge the possible embarrassment on both sides. The handout may be photocopied for this purpose and freely distributed to patients and clients.

As women are educated about breast examination, they should also be encouraged to inform their partners, husbands or brothers about TSE. It could also be taught to prospective fathers attending antenatal classes for lessons in parenting skills.

It is interesting to note that recent research has showed that the majority of men questioned had heard about TSE through the mass media and various instructional material; none of them had heard it from a nurse (Blesch, 1986). Information about TSE can be therefore very successfully spread through television or radio programmes and articles could be presented to local newspapers and magazines. Leaflets should be also made available in waiting rooms of hospitals, GPs' surgeries, health centres and public places like libraries. A small pamphlet on TSE could be included into condom packs.

Many recent health campaigns have focused around the early detection of women's diseases (eg, breast and cervical cancer). Men must also be involved in their own health screening and made aware that they are not immune from disease. Committed education programmes to inform men about testicular cancer and efficacy of TSE could save many lives at the moment being needlessly lost.

References
Blesch, K.S. (1986) Health beliefs about testicular cancer and self-examination among professional men. *Oncology Nursing Forum*, **13**, 1, 29–33.
Carlin, P.J. (1986) Testicular self-examination: A public awareness program. *Public Health Reports*, **101**, 1, 98–102.
Conklin, M. *et al* (1978) Should health teaching include self-examination of the testis? *American Journal of Nursing*, **78**, 12, 2073–4.
Davies, J.M. (1981) Testicular cancer in England and Wales. *The Lancet*, **1**, 928–32.
Forrester, D.A. (1986) Myths of masculinity: Impact upon men's health. *Nursing Clinic North America*, **21**, 15–23.
Ganang, L.H. *et al* (1987) Young men's knowledge of testicular cancer and behavioural intentions towards testicular self-examination. *Patient Education Counselling*, **9**, 3, 251–61.
Thornhill, J.S. *et al* (1986) Public awareness of testicular cancer and the value of self-examination. *British Medical Journal*, **293**, 480–1.

Useful addresses
For further educational material of TSE contact:
1. Yorkshire Regional Cancer Organisation, Cookridge Hospital, Leeds LS16 6QB.
For a video demonstrating TSE, price £7.50 per copy.
2. Leaflets on TSE can be ordered free (up to 250 copies) from:
Mr Evan Urquhart, Senior Project Manager, McCormick Ltd, Church House, Church Square, Leighton Buzzard LU7 7AE.

Handout: testicular self-examination

As we are all responsible for our own health and wellbeing, we need to learn how to care for our own bodies and how to detect early abnormalities. Testicular cancer is a relatively rare disease, mainly affecting men between the age of 15 and 40 years. If the cancer is diagnosed and treated at an early stage, the cure rate is almost 100 per cent. Yet, if diagnosis is delayed it can be a fatal illness.

Monthly testicular examination is a simple procedure you yourself can do. If you find anything abnormal it isn't necessarily cancerous – there are many other conditions affecting the testicles – but it is important that you consult your doctor.

How to examine your testicles

1. Examine yourself on the first day of each month so you remember easily.
2. Following a warm bath or shower (the scrotum is then 'relaxed' and easier to examine) look at your scrotum in front of a mirror. The left side of the scrotum usually hangs lower than the right.
3. Feel the weight and size of each testicle.
4. Roll each testicle gently between your thumb and fingers (Figure 1).

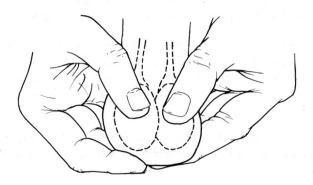

Figure 1. Roll each testicle gently between finger and thumb.

5. Locate the epididymis, which is a cord-like structure a the back of your testicle. It is always slightly tender when pressed. The spermatic cord extends upwards from the epididymis (Figure 2).
6. It will take a while to become confident in doing this self-examination.

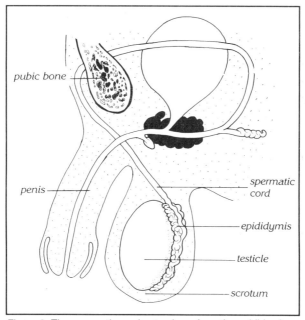

Figure 2. The spermatic cord extends up from the epididymis.

Contact your doctor:
- If you can only feel one testicle if your scrotum (men with undescended testicles are at slightly greater risk of getting testicular cancer).
- If your scrotum is slightly enlarged and you have a feeling of dragging and heaviness. (Pain is experienced by very few patients).
- If you have noticed a small lump or irregularity on the testicle.
- If you are simply unsure about how to examine yourself.

Remember:
If you notice anything unusual, it isn't necessarily cancerous. But don't delay in consulting your doctor; only he can make the final diagnosis.

Further information
For more information on testicular cancer, contact:
1. BACUP, 121/123 Charterhouse Street, London EC1M 6AA. (Tel: 071-608 1661).
2. SOS (Save Our Sons), Shirley Wilcose, 1 Rite Hill, Wootton Bridge, Isle of Wight PO33 4LA.
3. Yorkshire Regional Cancer Organisation, Cookridge Hospital, Leeds LS16 6QB.

29

Adolescents: alone together

Stevie Miller SRN, RSCN, RCNT

Paediatric Nurse Teacher, Southampton University College of Nursing and Midwifery

Most paediatric units care for children with a variety of medical and surgical problems encompassing the age range of birth to sixteen. Although the wards may be divided into different specialties as well as age groups, it has been of concern for some time that the problem of specific provision for the needs of adolescents was not being addressed.

In 1979 the Court Report indicated that it had been increasingly evident, in recent years, that adolescents presented with needs and problems which were sufficiently different from those experienced by children or adults and that adolescents required consideration as a distinct group for health care provision. In recognising the potential needs of this client group, The National Association Of the Welfare Of Children In Hospital (NAWCH) in 1990 published guidelines outlining standards of care for adolescents in hospital.

Defining adolescence

How can adolescence be defined? Three possible approaches have been considered by Kuykendall (1989). The first is to categorise an adolescent by chronological age. The problem this presents is the conflicting views expressed by authors in their statement as to when this period begins and ends. Some argue that the age range is from 12–19 years and others that it is from 13–20 years. It would thus appear that the period encompassing adolescence is not fixed and therefore chronological age is not a viable approach if taken in isolation.

The second approach which expands on the chronological model of adolescence is that of social status acquisition. This states that at various chronological ages individuals gain additional social privileges and status which may then be used to define the stage of life they have reached. Such an approach can certainly be viewed as being created by society according to society's arbitrary needs, eg lack of employment or insufficient manpower (Mackenzie, 1988).

The third approach to defining adolescence is that of the development theory. This characterises adolescence by what is happening socially, intellectually, emotionally, physically, sexually and psychologically. Using this approach adolescence can be divided into early, middle and late stages according to the behaviour patterns exhibited by the individual.

Developmental changes during adolescence

Physical development   Physical development in the adolescent is of great importance, not only for its own sake but for its emotional and social implications (Mackenzie, 1988). Coleman (1984) suggests that adolescents have two main body images: the way they think they look ie their body image, and the way they would like to look or their ideal body image. These self-perceptions are extremely important and are increasingly so when hospital admission threatens to make the gap between these two images even wider. Denholm (1985) cites studies implying that any impairment of body image may have significant consequences at this time. He uses the situation of immobilisation, and its resultant containment of impulsivity and reduction of independence, as an example.

Emotional and social development   During this time the emotional and social development is also significant. It is a time of potential stress for all parties involved where the young person seeks to find their own identity, ideals and place in society.

Erikson (1974) has identified the central problem of early adolescence as establishing a sense of 'who am I' and a preoccupation with how they are viewed by others. They are also concerned with society's expectations of them. Erikson suggests that failure to find this sense of identity results in identity diffusion or 'dropping out'.

Young people in 'primitive' cultures may be required to undergo rituals that formerly signify the end of childhood and the commencement of an adult role. Although this would appear to limit choice, it could present a form of security for an adolescent that may be lacking within the supposed freedom of our society.

Weller (1985) describes the developmental 'tasks' of adolescence as forming a clear individual identity.

- attaining emancipation from parents and developing a personal value system;
- achieving financial and social independence.
- developing relationships with members of both sexes.
- developing cognitive skills and the ability to think abstractly.
- developing the ability to control behaviour according to socially acceptable norms.
- taking responsibility for one's behaviour.

The term 'identity' encompasses four basic aspects of personality. These include:

- personal identity (where there is development of an individual perspective and direction in preparation for adulthood.
- continuity of personal character making a meaningful link between the end of childhood and aspirations for the future.
- the combination of physical development and social influences in the growth of the ego. According to Freud (1953) ego is that part of the

personality suppressed until it can be expressed in socially acceptable ways.

● The fourth basic aspect is that of solidarity with the ideals and identity of the peer group. This may lead to over-identification with individuals within the peer group who are particularly admired by the adolescent.

Adolescents need to seek comfort from, and test the loyalty of, members of their group in order to help each other through all the discomfort and uncertainty caused by the bodily changes, as well as the choices and conflicts presented by approaching adulthood.

With maturing cognitive processes, a child's thinking is no longer solely concerned with what is seen and heard, or based in the present. Adolescents are capable of imagining the conditions of an abstract problem, be it in the past, present or future. They can accept hypotheses and draw appropriate conclusions. With this development of reasoning comes the questioning of religious and political views and the challenging of parental attitudes and behaviour. The volatile and impulsive responses often demonstrated by adolescents with their tendency to challenge or defy authority, are all factors that may often be viewed as disturbing. All these however, are part of the adolescent's struggle to establish and maintain a growing sense of independence.

Unfortunately, opportunities are often lost in school, in the family and within our society for giving them a healthy self-image and enabling them to realistically and constructively view themselves as valuable members of the community contributing at both individual and social levels. Because of the scattering of this age group throughout a district hospital, health care professionals may also be losing valuable opportunities to meet this client group's specific health education needs.

Meeting adolescents' health needs

If it is accepted that adolescents do form a distinct client group, how can their needs best be met? Some 40 years ago it was usual for children of all ages to be cared for on adult wards. It was recognised by some nursing and medical staff at the time that children, especially those below the age of three years, required separate accommodation and facilities to cater for their quite different care needs. It may be argued that the position is the same now with regard to adolescents as it was with the under threes previously.

Young individuals with chronic conditions such as diabetes, cystic fibrosis and asthma, on reaching adolescence no longer feel comfortable in the environment of the children's ward they are likely to have frequented over the years. The atmosphere is often no longer conducive to them even though the primary members of the medical and nursing team may have remained constant.

Crying babies and generally noisy surroundings are now far less tolerable even though the adolescents will admit that, given the opportunity, they would generate plenty of noise themselves, but of a different type.

At the same time, adolescents do not like being nursed on an adult ward where the patients are generally much older. If nursed in a cubicle on such a ward, they feel isolated from the day-to-day events with no-one to talk to.

Gordon (1981) suggests that the reasons for the slow provision of adolescent facilities within the country's district hospitals may be due in part to the professional groups involved. Nurses on adult wards may enjoy the enlivening influence of this age group on their wards, while physicians and surgeons may think that the suggestion of adolescent wards by paediatricians is an attempt to extend their influence because of lower bed occupancy resulting from a lower birth rate and better child health. He further proposes that if some of the empty accommodation on the children's wards was converted into specialised facilities for adolescents, more beds on adult wards would be free.

Adolescents can be considered to be the healthiest age group in the population yet there are a considerable number in hospital at one time, scattered among various specialties. Surgical patients outnumber medical, the most common surgical problems being acute abdominal conditions and tonsillectomies. Medical conditions include mainly those with diabetes, asthma, acute chest infections, viral meningitis and urinary tract infections. Congenital malformations are featuring less by this age. Adolescents figure largely in road accident statistics. Drug overdoses, particularly among girls, also seems to be a common problem in this age group (Gordon, 1981).

Should special units be provided?

In 1959 when the Platt Report made its original recommendations, the UK was experiencing a significant increase in the adolescent population following the post-war baby boom. The current relevance of this report needs to be viewed in light of the present falling numbers of adolescents, the increased sophisticated of young people and the developments in nursing. A changing picture is giving adolescents more opportunity to meet and relate with people of all ages so they no longer function exclusively within their own peer groups. Should special units therefore be provided for adolescents in hospitals?

Blunden (1989) suggests that consideration of demographic and cultural changes, as well as the wishes of the client group, should be taken before coming to any decisions. Pollock and Fry (1986) estimate that 8.3% of the population are aged between ten and fifteen years. Blunden states that in her healthy authority of Kettering there are approximately 22,443 people aged between eleven and sixteen years, but that this number is falling. She further indicates that there are 4,193 sixteen year olds and 3,240 eleven year olds, a drop which reflects national demographic trends. She feels, however, that in spite of this fall there are sufficient adolescents to merit a special unit. The results of a questionnaire by Blunden asking adolescents themselves where they would choose to be nursed was that a large proportion opted for care within adolescent units or children's wards although almost half of those aged thirteen years or older saw the adult ward as the more appropriate alternative to adolescent units.

In answering the question of which nurses are likely to have a sufficient knowledge of adolescence gained from their basic training, Blunden suggests that, on examining the syllabuses for registered nurse training, the Registered Nurse Mental Handicap (RNMH) nurses are the best qualified apart from the Registered Sick Children's Nurses (RSCN) who generally choose to work on paediatric wards, so not benefiting the 84% of adolescents being nursed on adult wards by Registered General Nurses. Because of the reality of the situation, the practical experience that RGNs have would appear to be the best.

Mitigating against adolescent units is the reality that the work can be hard, stressful and occasionally dangerous. This age group en masse can be threatening, staffing mix and levels would need to be thoroughly researched before contemplating the building of such a unit.

There is much evidence supporting the need for adolescent units and NAWCH standards for adolescents in hospital add weight to this by referring to most recent reports by the World Health Organisation. Current guidelines issued by the Department of Health recommend that adolescents are cared for by appropriately trained staff in separate areas designed to meet their needs. In spite of this, NAWCH currently estimate that between 50–70% of adolescents are placed inappropriately in adult wards.

The NAWCH review also states that the British Paediatric Association estimates a need for fifteen adolescent beds for each district general hospital serving a population of approximately 200,000. Whilst indicating that separate facilities in a self-contained unit is desirable, where this is not immediately possible, operating policies and facilities should take into account this age group's special needs and provide an area within the children's ward specifically set-aside for them. Other countries such as Finland, and notably the United States, have well-established adolescent services.

Addressing adolescents specific health needs
One area that could be said to be meeting the needs of the adolescent client group is the adolescent unit for sufferers from cystic fibrosis. This unit is within the Hospital for Sick Children, Belfast and consists of colour coordinated single bedrooms with lounge and kitchen facilities. Elsewhere, in adolescent units such as that within the Hospital For Sick Children, Toronto, there is provision made for the pursuit of appropriate leisure activities in addition to catering for this age group's increasing need for privacy.

In the UK, there are now a number of units catering for adolescents with acute medical and surgical conditions for example Wexham Park Hospital, Slough; St Mary's Hospital, Manchester and Bristol Children's Hospital.

Many of the factors outlined here have implications for the way in which future provision of adolescent care is perceived in the 1990s and this provision should reflect the imminent challenges of consumer-lead care with the implementation of the White Paper.

References

Blunden, R. (1989) Adolescence: 'An artificial state'. *Paediatric Nursing*, March, 12–13.

Coleman, J.C. (1984) *The Nature of Adolescence*, 3rd edn. Methuen, London.

Court Report (1976) *Committee On Child Health Services: Fit for the Future*, HMSO, London.

Denholm, C. (1985) Hospitalization and the adolescent patient: A review and some critical questions. *Journal of the Association For The Care Of Children's Health*, **13**, 109–15.

Erikson, E.H. (1974) Identity, Youth and Crisis, 2nd edn. W.W. Norton, New York.

Freud, S. (1953) *Three Essays On The Theory Of Sexuality*. Hogarth, London.

Gordon, R.R. (1981) The adolescent in hospital. *Nursing*, **24**, 1048–50.

Kuykendall, J. (1989) Adolescence: teenage trauma. *Nursing Times*, **85** (27), 26–8.

Mackenzie, H. (1988) Teenagers in hospital. *Nursing Times*, **84** (32), 58–61.

National Association For the Welfare Of Children In Hospital: Quality Review Series (1990). *Setting Standards For Adolescents In Hospital*. NAWCH, London.

Platt Report (1959) *The Welfare Of Children In Hospital: Platt's Report of the Committee on Child Health Services*. HMSO, London.

Pollack, M. and Fry, J. (1986) *Commonsense Paediatrics*. McGraw Hill, Maidenhead.

Swanwick, M. and Oliver, R.W. (1985) *Psychological Adjustment In Adolescence*. Bailliere Tindall, (1179–81), London.

Weller, B. (1985) *Paediatric Nursing, Practice and Techniques*. Harper and Row, London.

30

Behavioural disorders in adolescence

Stuart Gemmell, RMN

Community Therapist (Nurse), Brookvale Adolescent Service, Southampton

The term 'behavioural disorders in adolescence' is by definition a vast, complicated and multifarious minefield.

"Conduct disorders, sometimes called externalizing disorders, are characterized by severe and persistent antisocial behaviour. They form the largest single group of psychiatric disorders in older children and adolescence. The prevalence of conduct disorders is difficult to estimate because the dividing line between them and normal rebelliousness is arbitrary "(Gelder *et al*, 1989).

As this statement indicates the difficulty lies within the adolescent process which we generally accept to mean adolescents showing, by behavioural demonstration, the ambiguity, conflict and emotional turmoil that they may be experiencing inside. The conflict and possible turmoil may exist due to relationships with peers, parents, school, expectations and sexuality.

Some of the more severe behavioural disorders will be clarified, concentrating not on generalised behavioural mannerisms of youth, but on self destructiveness and systematic disruptional disorders that some adolescents feel they need to demonstrate in order to create change. Some of the current therapeutic tools being offered to those adolescents will then be highlighted.

Adolescence as a time of change

Adolescence is a time of change, loosely described as the period of growth between puberty and adulthood.

"Adolescence refers to the period of transition from childhood to adulthood. Its age limits are not clearly specified, but extends roughly from age 12 to the late teens, when the physical growth is nearly complete" (Hilgard *et al*, 1979).

During this period a time of conflict arises which can conveniently be described as a 'triad composition', those areas involved being the 'self', 'peers' and 'family'.

Problems with behaviour of adolescents   Behaviour problems are often described by parents whose children have entered their adolescent 'phase'. Such displays are well documented by the main media outlets. An example of which is the television series *Butterflies* in which Wendy Craig is often caught in the position of go-between for her husband and their two sons. Likewise, an article in *Good Housekeeping* describes vividly the range of behaviours in which some teenagers can entangle themselves and their parents. Colin Dunne (1990) delivers in the article a damning statement on youth and then goes on to describe his experience of his own adolescent children: ". . . The first thing you've got to remember is that sometime between the age of 12 and 20 young people resign from the human race. My three were about average teens. Number one took to her room and played deafening rock music for the next four years. In the time she spoke not a single civil word to anyone of voting age. Occasionally she would descend to say how much she hated (a) people who told her what to do, and (b) people who didn't tell her what to do. She'd then slam a few doors with hinge-smashing violence and storm back upstairs".

To a lesser or greater degree most adolescents display the above, as well as not washing, not changing clothes, not helping with household chores, or not attending school on a regular basis, treating the place like a hotel and generally being obstreperous, obstructive and obstinate. It is then little wonder that both adolescent and parents are exhausted by the hormonal changes let alone the emotional ones that the adolescent process throws up.

Behavioural disorders

Putting aside this overwhelming development and deluge of typical adolescent behaviour, we need to clarify the severe behavioural disorders. All such disorders have similar characteristics which include:

- a prolonged existence of the disorder.
- the disorder makes the adolescent and his or her family feel isolated and trapped.
- confusion exists on how, why and when the behavioural disorder came into being.
- the disorder has a hidden agenda which for the adolescent may include: guilt, anger and punishment of self and others.

In essence the key words which are attributed to behavioural disorders include guilt, lack of self-worth, low self-esteem and anger.

Adolescent behavioural disorders are not necessarily family centred. However, Snell in 1983 concluded the following: "The adolescent's relationship with his family can be very difficult. Teenagers are often hostile, argumentative and rebellious, particularly towards their parents. The reasons for this are easy to understand. On the one hand a young person is expected to be a man and become independent and on the other to be guided and controlled by his parents . . . . He needs his parents, but wants to break away from them. These opposing emotions make him angry and the anger is usually directed at his parents."

Causal factors

Before presenting the two main strands of behavioural disorders, a comment needs to be included addressing the possible causal factors of such disorders. This is rendered almost impossible due to the complexity of adolescence in that, throughout the turbulent period, anything and everything to varying degrees can add or subtract to both minor and major prolonged behavioural disorders. Likewise, the term delinquency is not given any substantial space due to its subjectivity, but, very broadly, adolescent behavioural disorders can be separated into two distinct strands, ie self-directed (self-harm) disorders, and externally directed (systematic influencing) disorders. The Oxford Dictionary defines a system as: "a complex whole; a set of connected things or parts; an organised body or material or immaterial things". There is an argument to suggest that all behavioural disorders are systemic influencing. However, the distinction should be made between the internalised anger, and the externalised anger of punishing self and others.

Self-harm   The term 'self-harm' in adolescents has been the umbrella phrase given to adolescents who self-mutilate (wrist-cutting), self-poison (overdosing, solvent abuse) and go on to include anorexia, all of which can become prolonged, entrenched disorders affecting the adolescent. There are, of course, other forms of self-harm which can include running away from home and sexual promiscuity.

These behavioural disorders often occur in young people who suffer low self-esteem and feelings of rejection, frequently feeling they do not get the attention they want or indeed require from significant people around them. Why this should happen is the subject of continuing debate.

Acting-out   Externalised behavioural disorders are by design much more obvious and pronounced. Often described as 'acting out', the externalised behavioural umbrella often includes being verbally and physically aggressive, stealing, and disruption to family, school and community life.

The adolescent caught up in the above activity may similarly suffer from lack of self-worth, poor self-esteem and lack of respect for self and others. Viewed externally it can be seen that not only are parents, siblings and other significant persons suffering hurt and pain, but also the adolescents themselves.

The obvious biological changes which occur in adolescence are accompanied by an awareness of one's own sexuality. The emergence of this can be frightening, bewildering and overwhelming, such feelings often present themselves by means of hostility (verbal or physical).

Therapeutic interventions

It is within the triad composition of conflict between self, peer and family that most therapeutic interventions are delivered. Experience has shown that unless the adolescents themselves acknowledge a 'difficulty', little headway is going to be made. When dealing with adolescents within the psychiatric services one should establish how the adolescent views his or her referral. The reason for this concern is that many individuals in society have difficulty with the label 'psychiatry' and this will need to be acknowledged particularly as this is prevalent in adolescents.

Individual therapy   Nearly all adolescents attending an adolescent psychiatric service will be seen individually. For the majority of these adolescents, it is an opportunity for the therapist to clarify how the adolescent sees his or her world and may be nothing short of assessing how he or she views things. This might be a one-off assessment session. Some individuals may see a therapist on a regular basis who is able to facilitate, through a trust rapport, expression of some of the adolescent's gravest concerns and experiences. There is no fixed time span to this but some services go through a form of 'contracting' process, whereupon a set number of sessions are negotiated and once completed are either repeated or finished by means of a review and evaluation process.

The benefits of seeing adolescents on an individual basis are that the therapist will be non-judgmental and objective and the adolescent is given the opportunity to learn through trust the concepts of confidentiality, acceptance and self-worth. Disadvantages of this can include such things as dependence on the therapist, and using the therapist as a weapon against parents. The therapist's aims and objectives will be determined through the negotiated contractual relationship with the individual adolescent.

Peer group therapy   Most adolescent services offer group therapy sessions. In the 80s group therapy became highly valued, and now not only are they available within the health services but many nurses are involved in offering peer group therapy to other agencies. An article by Duncan Tennant (1988) adequately describes the rationale behind peer group therapy:

1. "Socialising techniques can be learned much more effectively in a group. The open feedback it gives participants can highlight nuances and mannerisms, which, unknown to them, have been undermining their relationships".

2. "We all live, work and play in groups. Whether or not your social needs are met is largely determined to our ability to function with others, yet there is no acceptable way of examining and working on group relations. A therapeutic group offers just that opportunity."

Tennant further states that peer group therapy is a good learning ground with feedback on how others view us. Any adult knows from personal experience as an adolescent that peers have as much influence as parents, teachers, etc.

One of the many positive factors is the self-help nature of many adolescent groups, where upon the adolescent supports his or her peers whilst at the same time receiving support.

In addition there can be many negative factors and the following may occur. Adolescents have the wonderful, yet damning, ability to recognise and expose other people's Achilles heel, and this can often result in scapegoating of individuals within the group.. Secondly there is the inability of some adolescents to share their feelings with their peers. Finally, many adolescents are quite fragile, despite 'cool' exteriors, and exposure to such peer group dynamics may be the very 'excuse' they need to scurry back to their own shell-like existence. This causes complications which make the setting-up of peer groups extremely difficult.

Family therapy   If one interchanges the term 'system' with family, then it becomes self-evident that an adolescent does affect the system he or she is in. Likewise, much of the other systemic activity (ie, parent's marital relationship, work, family/systemic communication) affects the adolescent. Family therapy is proving to be an effective means of dealing with behavioural disorders in adolescents.

One of the forerunners of family therapy and systemic thinking is Salvador Minuchin (1983). He offers insight not only into systemic processes but also into the nature of adolescent behavioural problems. The following extracts illustrate some of the many examples Minuchin gives in his text:

1. "One of most common precipators is the emergence of a child into adolescence. At that time the child's participation in the extrafamilial world and his status in that world increase. The relationship between child and parents is dislocated. The adolescent should be moved a little away from the sibling subsystem and given increased autonomy and responsibility appropriate to his age."

2. "At the time of therapy, the relationship of the mother and oldest son is fraught with his demands for autonomy, countered by her demands for obedience."

Most of the behavioural problems that adolescents present with are ventilated within their family. It is therefore necessary and highly appropriate that much of the therapeutic work carried out is directed towards the family. The more communication the therapist facilitates the greater the understanding parents have of the difficulties and changes their adolescents are facing, and the greater the awareness the adolescents have in hearing what struggles their parents have with dealing or even understanding their plight. It must be remembered, however, that sometimes families are so entrenched and enmeshed that increasing family communication is a non-starter.

Growing-up pains
Some of the difficulty arising from exploring this subject stems from the

fact that adolescents express themselves through behavioural means rather more successfully than in verbal ways. The added difficulties have been that behaviour is a continuum that is often misinterpreted and when writing or reading about adolescents one becomes flooded or twinged with memories of one's own adolescent history. With all these thoughts in mind, the area of behavioural disorders in adolescents is not necessarily best described by the medical profession but rather more poignantly, and certainly more humourously, in the arts. Two such books are by J. D. Salinder and S. Townsend.

In his book, *The Catcher in the Rye,* Salinger describes with alarming insight the difficulties that many adolescents often experience. Often witty, dreadfully sad, and sometimes confusing, Salinger opens his book with the following comments from the leading character Holden Caulfield: "If you really want to hear about it, the first thing you'll probably want to know is where I was born, and what my lousy childhood was like, and how my parents were occupied and all before they had me, and all that David Copperfield kind of crap, but I don't feel like going into it . . . Besides, I'm not going to tell you my whole goddam autobiography or anything. I'll just tell you about this madman stuff that happened to me around last Christmas before I got pretty rundown and had to come out here and take it easy."

The second author, Townsend in her book *The Secret Diary of Adrian Mole Aged 13¾,* writes about a delightful character named Adrian Mole. Equally with brilliant insight, Townsend delivers the plight of an adolescent to her readers in humourous yet all too familiar fashion. "Friday January 2nd. I felt rotten today. It's my mother's fault for singing 'My Way' at two o'clock in the morning at the top of the stairs. Just my luck to have a mother like her . . . The spot on my chin is getting bigger, it's my mother's fault for not knowing about vitamins."

Throughout the diary Adrian anguishes over the dawning realisation that his parents are not the all knowing, all loving creatures he once thought. "Saturday February 7th. My mother and father have been shouting at each other non-stop for hours. It started because of the bacon down the side of the fridge and carried on into how much my father's car is costing to repair. I went to my room and put my Abba records on. My father had the nerve to crash open and ask me to turn the volume down. I did. When he got downstairs I turned it up again."

The recommendation therefore is not to get too bogged down in psychiatric textbooks dealing with adolescent disorders, but to enjoy the wealth of books dealing with 'growing-up pains'.

Both books highlight the dilemmas that both characters face, while also giving insight into the behaviourisms employed by adolescents in expressing their emotions. Finally, behavioural displays are to be expected, indeed appropriate, from all adolescents. They only become disorders when they are prolonged, immobilise the adolescent and his or her family from daily activity, become life threatening and finally become intolerable in their management.

References
Dunne, C. (1990) *Good Housekeeping*. IPC magazines, London.
Gelder, Gath and Mayou (1989) *Oxford Textbook of Psychiatry*, 2nd edn. Oxford Medical Publications, Oxford.
Hilgard, Atkinson and Atkinson (1979) *Introduction to Psychology*, 7th edn. Harcourt Brace Jovanovich, USA.
Minuchin, S. (1983) *Families and Family Therapy*. Tavistock Publications, London.
Salinger, J. D. (1979) *The Catcher in the Rye*. Penguin Modern Classics, Penguin, Harmondsworth.
Snell, H. (1983) Mental Disorders: An Introductory Book for Nurses. George Allen & Unwin, London.
Tennant, D. (1988) Classroom Psychiatry. *Nursing Times*, **84** (7).
Townsend, S. (1984) The Secret Diary of Adrian Mole Aged 13¾ Methuen, London.

Bibliography
Erikson, E. H. (1968) *Identity Youth and Crises*. Norton, New York.
Argyle, M. (1979) *The Psychology of Interpersonal Behaviour*, 3rd edn. Pelican, London.
Rutter, M. (1975) *Helping Troubled Children*. Penguin, Harmondsworth.
Bettelheim, B. (1959) *Love is Not Enough*. Free Post, USA.

Hospitals and Illness: A Child's Perspective

31

Its OK having asthma . . . young children's beliefs about illness

Christine Eiser, BSc (Hons), PhD

Senior Research Fellow, Department of Psychology, Washington Singer Laboratories, University of Exeter

Children's knowledge of and attitudes towards health and illness change with age. It is important for health professionals to understand these changes if they are to communicate successfully with children about their illness and treatment, and to realise that each child's development is unique and cannot be rigidly categorised.

Why understand children's views?

Health education All children need to develop positive attitudes to self-care and health behaviour; partly for their own immediate benefit and partly because such habits are likely to promote positive healthcare behaviour in adulthood. For example, attitudes toward smoking develop early, and early tobacco use appears to increase the likelihood that illegal drugs will be used in later adolescence. Positive adult attitudes to dental care can be promoted by health education in the young (Eiser, 1989).

Hospital admission for acute illness Children seem to suffer less stress associated with short-term hospital admission when they are given information about their treatment and what to expect.

Chronic disease Children with chronic diseases (eg, epilepsy, diabetes, asthma) are often encouraged to become responsible for many aspects of their treatment. It is therefore necessary to explain what needs to be done; when, how and why.

Given the range of situations in which effective communication about illness is necessary, much research has centred on what illness means to young children. There appear to be age-related changes in beliefs about illness: older children explain illness in more complex terms, refer more frequently to internal body cues, are more focused on specific diseases and can better describe process and cause (Bibace and Walsh, 1981).

More specifically it has been argued that children under seven years of age tend to believe illnesses are a punishment for wrong-doing, occur by some magical process, or towards the end of the age-period, are 'caught' from others. From seven to 11 years, they believe illnesses are contracted through contact with germs, and it is not until approximately 11 years of age that they understand enough about their bodies to realise that illnesses can also result from a failure of some specific body part.

These results have been taken to imply that children go through a series of stages in their beliefs about illness, and that these stages parallel those described by Piaget to account for development in physical concepts, such as space or time. A corollary of this approach is that children need a certain kind of explanation of illness which is 'matched' to their cognitive level, and will be unable to understand more advanced explanations. Thus, the seven-year-old is likely to understand the cause of illness if this is explained in terms of contagion, but will not understand a physiologically based explanation. There is, however, a danger in over-interpreting these findings and being too rigid in giving explanations to children.

There are both methodological and theoretical difficulties in the interpretation of this work. Methodologically, researchers often use prolonged and unnatural questioning with children; there is little comparability across studies in the kinds of questions asked, and work is invariably based only on small samples of healthy children. Theoretically, there has been no adequate explanation of how children shift from one stage to the other, nor of the role of emotions or personal experience in determining children's explanations. It is perhaps this lack of awareness of how experience affects children's understanding that has been especially damning to the stage approach.

Children's knowledge   Given these criticisms, our research in this field (Eiser, Eiser and Lang, 1989) was based on a model that emphasises what the child knows and the role of the experience. According to 'script' theory (Nelson, 1986) children learn through participation in routine everyday events, so the study began by asking 20 children from two age groups (five and eight years) "What happens when you go to the doctor (or dentist, or hospital)?". All the children attended the same small primary school and there were equal numbers of boys and girls in each group. The conversations with the children took place immediately before the whole school embarked on a project about health and illness.

Children of both age groups were able to give well-ordered accounts of the sequence of events involved, ie they organised their descriptions according to the following sequence:

- **Cause** Some children discussed why the visit to the doctor/ dentist/hospital was necessary, or why they were unwell or needed an operation. These precursors to the main event were discussed in terms of symptoms ("I had toothache"; "My throat was sore") or accident ("I fell out of a tree").

- **Journey** Children may describe the journey to the surgery ("We take the bus into town"; "They wheel you along the corridor on a trolley").

- **Reception** This refers to the time spent in the waiting-room prior to seeing the doctor or dentist ("We wait outside and Mummy reads me a story"; "We wait till the nurse calls our name").

- **Inspection/diagnosis** This refers to the main diagnostic interview ("You open your mouth and the dentist looks inside with his mirror"; "Mummy tells the doctor what's wrong and he listens to your heart").

- **Treatment/cure** This refers to the treatment offered ("The dentist cleans your teeth"; "They take your tonsils out"; "You stay in bed and have some medicine").

- **End of treatment** This describes the acts that signal the end of the encounter with medical personnel, and occurred most frequently in the 'dentist' script ("The dentist gives you a sticker"; "We make an appointment for next time").

- **Journey home** ("We walk home"; "We go shopping and Mummy buys me a treat").

- **Recovery** ("When I'm better, I go back to school").

Ordering experiences

Children appear to organise their knowledge about hospitals and medical visits in terms of sequences of events, and this may well enable them to predict what will happen in future encounters, but this study was conducted with children of school age, and required them to verbalise their descriptions. In a further study, a picture-sequencing task was used to see if four-year-olds could also order their experiences (Eiser, Eiser and Jones, 1991).

Each child (n=90) was shown five photographs of hospital scenes. The scenes were made up from Playmobil toys and showed an ambulance, children eating on a hospital ward, children playing in a hospital ward, a surgery and a more formal scene where children were in hospital beds in rows, with less sign of ordinary games activities. The four-year-olds agreed on the ordering of the photographs: the ambulance was placed first, followed by the surgery, meal-times, formal ward scene and finally the less formal play scene. This implies that even young children without personal experience of hospital admission were aware that people go to hospital by ambulance, and are not allowed to eat until after surgery.

Half the children were then shown the informal play scene and the remainder the formal scene, and asked to look at it carefully for 10 seconds. They were then shown 12 photographs, each depicting one item. Four of these items had appeared in the original photograph (correct), four showed objects that might have been in a hospital scene but weren't on the photograph (plausible) and four showed items that would never be found in a hospital (implausible). The mean number of correct items was high (mean for formal scene = 3.27, informal = 3.11). More importantly, children were more likely to make plausible than implausible errors. Ignoring ties, 17 children chose more plausible than implausible items in the informal scene, and four chose more implausible. In the formal scene, 26 children chose more plausible items and none more implausible items. This suggests children even of this young age have well-developed beliefs about what happens in hospital, and that this allows them to make inferences about what they might see, rather than simply recall what was in the photograph.

Taken together, these data suggest that, from two years of age, children have well-ordered ideas about what hospital is like and what happens there, and that this information must be gained from such sources as television, books or other people's accounts, rather than their own experience. The fact that children have such information is both an advantage and disadvantage. It is an advantage to the extent that it allows them to make some predictions as to what hospital is like and what happens there; but a disadvantage if their experiences clash with these expectations. Children with serious or chronic diseases are especially likely to find that their experiences do not match expectations.

Children with chronic disease

Chronic diseases and their treatments can be particularly difficult for children to understand. Sometimes (as for children with leukaemia), they can feel quite well before a hospital appointment, but much worse afterwards. Treatments often continue for many years, and also require children to become increasingly responsible for their own health. Those with diabetes for example, must monitor their diets, test blood sugar levels and self-inject insulin. It is often difficult for children to understand why these tasks are necessary, and it is understandable, therefore, that some children perceive them as some kind of punishment. Despite careful explanations, some children with diabetes seem to feel that not being allowed to eat sweets is a punishment for eating far too many before their diagnosis. However, this emphasis on punishment is not necessarily the norm. In a study of 47 children with diabetes, 34 felt it was a 'good' thing, arguing that not being allowed to eat sweets meant that they were less likely to get fat or have spotty skin and more likely to have strong teeth compared with their 'healthy' friends (Eiser *et al*, 1988).

It is often difficult for adults to appreciate which aspects of a disease are the most difficult for a child to cope with. Given the range of aggressive and painful treatments experienced by children with leukaemia, for example, it is surprising to find that many feel that the relatively innocuous finger-prick is the worst thing that happens to them.

For the eight-year-old boy quoted left, having asthma means he might make a fool of himself in front of his class. He understands that his father had asthma as a child, but no longer suffers, and his knowledge results in a rather confused understanding that asthma can be shared around, more like a contagious disease than an inherited condition. There are other indications that children can feel shame or embarrassment about their condition. Colland (1988) for example, found that children described their asthma in the following ways: "I make high noises and everyone can hear me"; "I am ill and often wheezy"; "I cannot go to the zoo"; "I cannot have a dog"; "I am afraid to die"; "Other children tease me"; "I have to take stupid medicines every day". Asked how they managed to take medication at school, they replied:-"Quickly, so no-one can see"; "After everyone has left the classroom and gone outside"; "I don't take them"; "In the toilets so no-one can see".

It is one thing to explain a disease and its treatment to a child in terms of physiological processes; it is quite another to address issues of shame, guilt and embarrassment that can be associated with diagnoses.

A range of understanding

Children vary enormously in their abilities to understand illness and treatment, and this understanding is determined as much by their personal experience as any maturational process. Illness experience is in any case, very idiosyncratic. In the process of conducting research we recently asked eight-year-olds and 11-year-olds to tell us the names of all the illnesses they knew, expecting that the eight-year-olds at least would be limited to knowledge of childhood infectious diseases. Although this was true for a small percentage, the range of cited diseases was extremely wide. One child only knew about diseases contracted by horses! Others (who admitted to watching lots of television), knew about Aids, heart attacks and nervous breakdowns. Still others knew more about leprosy than anything else. The moral is that we should never assume a child's knowledge; they can be surprising both in terms of what they know and what they don't know.

Healthcare professionals must be more prepared to use a variety of methods to elicit children's knowledge, rather than rely on verbal questions and answers. Toys that are familiar to young children are specially useful.

We also need to be aware that increasing children's knowledge of illness is not necessarily a good thing, especially if the illness is chronic or life-threatening. Children who had greater awareness of diabetes have been found to be more distressed and anxious than those who were less well-informed (Allen *et al*, 1984). Making children more knowledgeable about their illness must, therefore, go hand-in-hand with a preparedness to tackle the social and emotional consequences of that knowledge. There is increasing evidence that it is emotional development, far more than the cognitive or intellectual, that is attenuated in sick children. Harris (1988) found that children hospitalised briefly for acute illness were less aware that emotional reactions could determine the course of recovery from an illness than age-matched healthy controls.

Children's beliefs about illness will be determined at least in part from those of their family. Among those with diabetes, children from poorly functioning families are likely to experience difficulties in compliance and haemoglobin control (Hauser *et al*, 1986). Children from families that function well are less likely to experience similar difficulties. Communications with children must take into account the beliefs and understanding about illness and treatment held by the child's whole family.

Finally, it is often assumed that from 11 to 12 years of age, children's knowledge and ability to understand information conforms increasingly to medical doctrine. Certainly, adolescents' biological knowledge becomes much more extensive (Carey, 1985), but there continue to be widely held myths and confusions over many issues. While the concern with how to improve communication with young children is welcome, it needs to be seen as part of a much wider issue. There is a continuing need to integrate medical knowledge within an individual's general framework for understanding illness. Within this perspective communicating with patients, whether children or adults, demands the treading of a delicate balance between the need to impart high technology information as quickly as possible with individual beliefs, drawn from a variety of sources over an extended period of time.

References

Allen, D.A., Affleck, G., Tennen, H., McGrade, G.J., Ratzan, S. (1984) Concerns of children with a chronic illness: a cognitive-developmental study of juvenile diabetes. *Child Care, Health and Development*, **10**, 211–18.

Bibace, R. and Walsh, M.E. (1981) Children's Conceptions of Health, Illness and Bodily Functions. Jossey-Bass, San Francisco.

Carey, S. (1985) Conceptual Change in Childhood. MIT Press, Cambridge, Mass.

Colland, B. (1988) Outwikkelings-psychologische aspectin by astma. *Kind en Adolescentie*, **9**, 85–97.

Eiser, C. (1989) Children's Concepts of Illness: Towards an alternative to the stage approach. *Psychology and Health*, **3**, 93–101.

Eiser, C., Eiser, J.R., and Jones, B.A. (1991) Scene schemata and scripts in children's understanding of hospital. *Child Care, Health and Development*, **16**, 303–13.

Eiser, C., Eiser, J.R., and Lang, J. (1989) Scripts in children's reports of medical events. *European Journal of Psychology of Education*, **IV**, 377–84.

Eiser, C., Swindell, A., Eiser, J.R., Penfold, J., Mann, L. (1988) Interviews with Diabetic Children. Flinders University of S. Australia, unpublished report.

Hauser, S. *et al* (1986) Children with recently diagnosed diabetes: Interactions within their families. *Health Psychology*, **5**, 273–96.

Nelson, K. (1986) Event Knowledge: Structure and Function in Development. Lawrence Erlbaum, New Jersey.

Acknowledgements

The author is supported by the ESRC, England.

32

What children think about hospitals and illness

Christine Eiser, BSc (Hons), PhD
Senior Research Fellow, Department of Psychology, Washington Singer Laboratories, University of Exeter

Despite the enormous improvements made in caring for sick and hospitalised children since the publication of the Platt report (1959), admission to hospital is still a traumatic event. It is particularly traumatic for young children, who are much less well-informed than adults about ward procedures and treatments. Preschool children in particular may hold quite unpredictable views about what happens in hospitals. Redpath and Rogers (1984) found that some children believed that you went to hospital healthy and became ill while there. This and other research (Eiser and Patterson, 1984) has shown that young children may think that people in hospital always die, or that admission to hospital lasts for years, rather than days or weeks.

Less dramatically, but just as important in terms of how children perceive hospitals, is their confusion about the role of medical staff. In particular, Brewster (1982) showed that young children believed that doctors and nurses deliberately set out to hurt them, and this view was held even more strongly by children with a history of admissions compared with those with only brief experiences.

Punishment

Children differ greatly from adults in their understanding about the cause of illness, its treatment and prevention. There is some evidence that children's thoughts about illness change as they develop. Below seven years of age they may think that illness is a punishment for bad behaviour, or some magical rite.

They commonly think that all illnesses are contagious, and this may lead them to be suspicious of other children in the ward, fearing that they may 'catch' other illnesses (Bibace and Walsh, 1980). They do not understand how treatment can make them better, understandably — why should oral medication or an injection in the arm make a leg feel better?

Explanation of illness to children under seven must also take account of the fact that they have very limited understanding of their bodies (Crider, 1981; Eiser and Patterson, 1983) — they may be aware only that they have a heart, brain, blood and bones inside them. Awareness of their function is also very simple — the heart is for loving and the brain for 'doing sums'.

Misconceptions

Children between seven and 11 years become slightly more sophisticated, though their views are still by no means adult. Illness is caused by contact with 'germs', and there is still the belief that illness is generally spread by contact with others. They do not correctly infer the reasons for treatment. Beuf (1979) found that it was often assumed that a return to a normal diet was a sign of relapse, rather than improvement. By 11 years of age, children know they have a stomach and lungs. The stomach is 'for storing food' and children may not reliably be aware that food is converted to blood and waste. Commonly, they may think they have only one lung, and that they breathe through the mouth.

Increasing sophistication and adult-like concepts emerge from 11 years of age. In particular, children become aware that illness can be aggravated by psychological factors, and that stress or anxiety can influence the course of a disease. They become aware of the connections within the body — that there are digestive, respiratory or circulatory systems for example. Of particular importance, they realise that treatment sometimes makes them feel worse rather than better, and that it may be necessary to endure short-term discomfort in the hope of longer-term cure.

Effect of experience

This approach to understanding how children think about illness should be seen as an approximate guide. Their beliefs are likely to be affected by individual experiences — some children with chronic diseases, for example, can become relatively mature in their understanding, especially of their own disease. Others, particularly young chronically ill patients, may see only that their illness results in parental anxiety. This, and the fact that doctors and parents tend to keep young patients uninformed about their illness to avoid causing them stress, may mean that they remain less sophisticated in their reasoning than healthy children who have little experience of hospitals (Eiser et al, 1984).

In answering paediatric patients' questions, it is important to be aware of the limitations of their knowledge, and that answers may be interpreted very differently from how they were intended. Many medical terms are easily misinterpreted by children, for example, a diagnosis of diabetes may be taken to mean that a child will 'die of betes'; a diagnosis of oedema that 'there is a demon in my belly' (Perrin and Gerrity, 1981). It is also helpful to realise that many young patients believe that all illnesses are contagious, since this is likely to influence their behaviour on the ward.

How else may the stress of hospitalisation be reduced for young children? Undoubtedly it is important that they have some idea as to what to expect on a hospital ward. Generally, attempts to prepare children before admission have been successful in reducing anxiety and/or improving ward behaviour. Many American hospitals provide preparation for children being admitted for routine surgery (Azarnoff and Woody, 1981). The most common methods involve the use of films or videos (Melamed and Seigel, 1975), home visits by nurses (Ferguson, 1979), play therapy (Cassell and Paul, 1967), or pre-admission tours (McGarvey, 1983). Unfortunately, most of this preparation is aimed at the child being admitted for routine surgery and there is little in the way of preparation offered to chronically sick children. It is easy to forget that however minor and routine the procedures may appear to staff, they are potentially very frightening for children. Clearly, it is impossible to provide preparation for children admitted following traumatic injury, so there has been a move to provide children in the general community with information, so that they have some idea about what to expect should they require admission to hospital (McGarvey, 1983). Tours of hospitals appear to be enjoyed by young children, though it is not known if they result in less trauma for those who are later admitted.

Nurses can do a lot to reduce the stress of a child's hospital admission. Play and educational facilities which provide a continuity between home and hospital life are important. In recognising that children have different concerns from adults and by being aware that they are ill-informed about hospital and treatment, the nurse may be better able to answer a child's questions appropriately.

Children are given very little information about their illnesses directly by medical staff (Pantell et al, 1982), and may have to glean knowledge from eavesdropping adult conversation. This inevitably leads to misunderstanding. It is important for all helath care professionals to appreciate the trauma hospital admission can cause to children and to ensure that they minimise its effect as much as possible.

References

Azarnoff, P. and Woody, P. (1981) Preparation of children for hospitalisation in acute care hospitals in the United States. *Pediatrics*, **68**, 361–8.

Beuf, A.H. (1979) *Biting off the bracelet: a study of children in hospital*. University of Pennsylvania Press, Philadelphia.

Bibace, r. and Walsh, M.E. (1980) Development of children's concepts of illness. *Pediatrics*, **66**, 913–17.

Brewster, A.B. (1982) Chronically ill hospitalised children's concepts of their illness. *Pediatrics*, **69**, 355–362.

Cassell, S. and Paul, M. (1967) The role of puppet therapy on the emotional responses of children hospitalised for cardiac catheterisation. *Pediatrics*, **71**, 233–39.

Crider, C. (1981) Children's concepts of the body interior. In: R. Bibace and M.E. Walsh (Eds.) *Children's conceptions of health, illness and bodily functions*. Jossey-Bass, San Francisco.

Eiser, C. and Patterson, D. (1983) "Slugs and snails and puppy-dog tail": children's ideas about the insides of their bodies. *Child: Care, Health and Development*, **9**, 233–40.

Eiser, C. and Patterson, D. (1984) Children's perceptions of hospital: a preliminary study. *International Journal of Nursing Studies*, **21**, 45–50.

Eiser, C., Patterson, D. and Tripp, J.H. (1984) Illness experience and children's conceptualisation of health and illness. *Child: Care, Health and Development*, **10**, 157–62.

Ferguson, B.F. (1979) Preparing young children for hospitalisation: a comparison of two methods. *Pediatrics*, **65**, 656–64.

McGarvey, M.E. (1983) Preschool hospital tours. *Children's Health Care*, **11**, 122–24.

Melamed, B.C. and Siegel, L.J. (1975) Reduction of anxiety in children facing hospitalisation and surgery by use of filmed modelling. *Journal of Consulting and Clinical Psychology*, **43**, 511–21.

Pantell, R.H., Stewart, T.J., Dias, J.K., Wells, P. and Ross, A.W. (1982) Physician communication with children and parents. *Pediatrics*, **70**, 396–402.

Perrin, E.C. and Gerrity, P.S. (1981) There's a demon in your belly. Children's understanding of illness. *Pediatrics*, **67**, 841–49.

Platt Committee, Great Britain (1959) *The Welfare of Children in Hospitals*. Her Majesty's Stationery Office, London.

Redpath, C. and Rogers, C.S. (1984) Healthy young children's concepts of hospitals, medical personnel, operations and illness. *Journal of Pediatric Psychology*, **9**, 29–40.

33

Preparing children for hospital: a school-based intervention

Christine Eiser, BSc (Hons), PhD
Senior Research Fellow, Department of Psychology, Washington Singer Laboratories, University of Exeter

Lesley Hanson, BA, RSCN, HVCert
School Nursing Sister, Exeter Health Authority

Hospital admission can be a frightening experience for children, particularly those who experience traumatic injury or sudden onset of chronic disease. To prepare them for the possibility of admission, it has been advocated that school-based education programmes be implemented (Elkins and Roberts, 1983; Peterson and Ridley-Johnson, 1983). This approach may also benefit children who are generally anxious about more routine visits to a doctor or dentist (Roberts et al, 1981).

One common approach to school-based intervention is the organised hospital tour. McGarvey (1983) reports that a programme for preschoolers, in which they were encouraged to "see, feel and experience" what happens in hospitals, was well received by children, teachers and parents. Three children who were subsequently hospitalised as emergency admissions were reported to adjust well.

An alternative technique involves setting up a 'play hospital' in school, and encouraging children to participate in both structured or free play situations (Brett, 1983). Elkins and Roberts (1984) set up a play hospital and used hospital volunteers dressed up as medical personnel to explain the equipment and procedures. The 25 children who took part in this activity subsequently reported fewer medical fears and were more knowledgeable about medical events than a control group of children.

Setting up a play hospital
This chapter is concerned with our own experiences in setting up a play hospital in primary schools, and describing the children's responses. The purpose of the study was twofold: to increase children's hospital related knowledge, and reduce anxiety and fear. Since some of the children were quite young, we did not feel verbally based assessments, such as interviews or questionnaires, were appropriate as the main techniques for evaluation. Instead, we focused on qualitative changes in the nature

of children's play. Groups of three children were videotaped playing with the equipment on two separate occasions, four weeks apart. During the intervening period, children were given the opportunity to handle and play with the equipment under the guidance of a school nurse and mother helpers. We hoped that, as a result of experience with the equipment and a range of educational activities, we would be able to identify changes in play, reflecting improved knowledge and attitudes towards hospitals and medical personnel.

Method

Subjects   The children all attended a small first school (catering for five- to eight-year-olds) in a rural Devon town. There is little local industry, and unemployment is relatively high. The school, like most others in the district, caters for children predominantly from working and lower middle-class homes. None of the children suffered from any chronic condition, or had personal experience of hospital other than as an outpatient. Subjects were drawn from the reception class (five to 5½ years) and the third and fourth year (seven to eight years). They were collected from the classroom in groups of three (normally same-sex triads), selected by the teacher. Selection was random, rather than in terms of friendship patterns or ability levels. In all, 14 triads of five-year-olds and eight triads of eight-year-olds took part in the study.

Apparatus   A miniature hospital was set up in an empty classroom in the school. It was divided into four areas.
- The **reception** area consisted of a table and two chairs opposite each other. On the table was a telephone, notepad and pencil. There was also a display rack containing a selection of health education leaflets.
- The **hospital ward** consisted of two beds made with blankets, and a baby's cot, complete with doll. There was a food table on one of the beds, and a 'drip' hanging at the side. On a small table nearby were several pairs of rubber gloves, cotton facemasks and head covers (of the type used in surgery). On a series of open shelves was an array of medical equipment, including a stethoscope, syringe, tweezers, respiratory mask and nursing bowls.
- In the **X-ray** area was a hard table covered with a sheet. Above the table was a pretend light that could be swung through a semicircle, and two X-rays were hung on the wall.
- In the **surgery** areas, another hard table was covered by a sheet. There was also another green sheet on top, with a hole through which the 'surgery' could be performed. On nearby shelves were a number of surgical overalls, hats, masks, gloves and overshoes. In addition, there was a set of surgical equipment.

We also had a selection of dressing-up clothes: nursing uniforms of several grades (dark blue for sister, light blue for staff nurse, green for students); a doctor's white coat, and various 'patient' outfits – pyjamas, nighties and dressing-gowns.

Procedure

The 'hospital' was set up in a spare classroom. Children were brought into the hospital in groups of three, and invited to play with the equipment for 10 minutes. Over the following month, a number of activities were organised. The children were brought back to the hospital on several occasions, by the school nurse and mother helpers. On these occasions, some of the equipment was pointed out, and ward and surgical procedures explained. Other activities included a visit to the children's ward at the local hospital, and visits to the school from an ambulance and crew, health visitor and a guide dog and owner. Each class also undertook a health-related group project.

At the second filming, children were again brought to the 'hospital' in groups of three (as before) and told that this was their last opportunity to play with the equipment before it was moved to another school. Again, their play was videotaped during the 10-minute session.

Results

Area of activity   During the first play session, most groups of children focused all their activities on the ward area, with only two groups using the surgery and one using X-ray equipment. During the second session, all groups organised their play throughout all areas of the hospital. Games were more sequenced – patients were 'admitted' to the ward, and subsequently moved to X-ray and surgery, before being discharged.

Use of equipment   Children used a range of equipment at both sessions, although at first the stethoscope, syringe, bandages and masks were used considerably more than other pieces of equipment. During the second session, there was much greater use of all the equipment, with less emphasis on the stethoscope and syringe. There were also differences in how the children used the equipment. During the first session, play was often quite rough. Children were quite aggressive in the way they gave injections, for example. On the second occasion, all children were considerably more gentle, and apparently more aware of the impact of treatment on the patient. 'Patients' were therefore likely to be warned that an injection might hurt.

'Healthcare staff' behaviour   There were substantial changes in the activities, particularly of nursing staff. During the first play session, nurses' activities involved care-taking, making beds, offering food and drink, or giving medicines. On the second, nurses spent a lot of time at the desk writing, or making phone calls. The role of the nurse seemed to have shifted from caretaker, to administrator!

Hospital atmosphere   On both occasions, children created an atmosphere of tension and emergency on the ward. Play invariably involved treating the very sick or dying, and speed and urgency characterised the interactions and conversations of staff.

Additional evaluations All the children greatly enjoyed their time in the play hospital, and were keen to participate. Eleven children were interviewed in depth about their reactions to the project, and asked to describe what they had learned. All appeared to have benefitted substantially, both in terms of special information acquired, and in the development of non-fearful attitudes to hospital.

Does the play hospital work?

The ultimate justification for school-based preparation for hospitalisation may well be that children are less anxious and fearful about admission. There are, however, many practical difficulties involved in such an evaluation, particularly in that there may be a long interval between the intervention and admission, and that other mediating factors might then determine the child's behaviour. Such arguments have been put forward, and along with financial cuts, resulted in a reduction in these activities (Azarnoff, 1982). Certainly, the changes we identified were short-term, and we cannot speculate on the long-term value of our intervention.

Even within the short-term, however, we feel we can point to some increase in children's hospital-related knowledge. At the second session, children's play reflected greater awareness of a range of medical equipment, as well as knowledge of activities typical of admission, X-ray and surgery, and ward procedures.

There were also changes in hospital-related attitudes. The children seemed to have gained empathy with the patient's role; nurses were careful to warn patients of impending pain. In this respect, children seemed to have acquired very realistic appraisals of what happens in hospital. They were not only more aware of different equipment and techniques, but also aware of the potentially painful nature of medical treatment.

Perhaps more unfortunate was the change in children's perceptions of the nurse's role. During the first play session, 'nurses' cared for patients and tried to make them comfortable. On the second 'nurses' were preoccupied with administrative tasks, and had little, if any, time left for patient care. There also appeared to be greater awareness of a hierarchy among staff, with junior nurses being subordinate to more senior staff. To some extent, this kind of play may be closer to reality than that shown prior to the intervention, nevertheless, it seems somewhat regrettable.

Given the potential stress associated with hospitalisation (Peterson and Ridley-Johnson, 1980), it is important to develop a range of preparatory techniques for children. The school-based educational programme appears to have considerable merit, not least because it can be made available to all children before the need arises. It is not altogether clear at what level the programmes are successful; whether by increasing hospital related knowledge, reducing anxiety or helping the child develop skills to cope with hospital procedures. The success of the latter, described as 'stress-inoculation' procedures (Zastowny et al, 1986) in reducing stress in other situations (public-speaking [Cradock et al, 1978], and dental treatment [Klingman et al, 1984]), attests to the potential value of this approach in preparing children for hospitalisation.

At a practical level, the success of the play hospital is probably as dependent on the energy and enthusiasm of staff and children as on the particular contents. The overriding feeling of those who took part, however, both adults and children, was that the experience was worthwhile, and everyone learned a lot.

References

Azarnoff, P. (1982) Hospital tours for school children ended. *Pediatric Mental Health*, 1, 2.

Brett, A. (1983) Preparing children for hospitalisation – a classroom teaching approach. *Journal of School Health*, 53, 561–63.

Craddock, C., Cotler, S., Jason, L.A. (1978) Primary prevention: Immunisation of children for speech anxiety. *Cognitive Therapy and Research*, 2, 389–396.

Elkins, R. and Roberts, M. (1983) Psychological preparation for pediatric hospitalisation. *Clinical Psychology Review*, 3, 275–295.

Elkins, P. and Roberts, M. (1984) A preliminary evaluation of hospital preparation for nonpatient children: Primary prevention in a 'Let's pretend hospital'. *Children's Health Care*, 13, 31–36.

Klingman, A., Melamed, B.G., Cuthbert, M.I., Hermecz, D.A. (1984) Effects of participant modelling on information acquisition and skill utilisation. *Journal of Consulting and Clinical Psychology*, 52, 414–422.

McGarvey, M.E. (1983) Preschool hospital tours. *Children's Health Care*, 11, 122–124.

Peterson, L. and Ridley-Johnson, R. (1980) Pediatric hospital response to survey a prehospital preparation for children. *Journal of Pediatric Psychology*, 5, 1–7.

Peterson, L. and Ridley-Johnson, R. (1983) Prevention of disorders in children. In Walker, C.E. and Roberts, M.C. (Eds.) *Handbook of Clinical Child Psychology*. Wiley-Interscience, New York.

Roberts, M.C., Wurtele, S.K., Boone, R.R., Ginther, L.J., Elkins, P.D. (1981) Reduction of medical fears by use of modelling: A preventive application in a general population of children. *Journal of Pediatric Psychology*, 6, 293–300.

Zastowny, T.R., Kirschenbaum, D.S., Meng, A.L. (1986) Coping skills training for children: Effects on distress before, during and after hospitalisation for surgery. *Health Psychology*, 5, 231–247.

Acknowledgments

This work was funded by the Nuffield Foundation. We would like to thank Miss Joan Cudmore and the staff and children of Cowleymoore First School, Devon, and Philip Gurr for technical assistance. James Lang assisted with some of the children's interviews.

34
Preparing children for hospital

Elizabeth M. Horne, MA
Publishing Director, Professional Nurse

Twenty five per cent of all children under the age of five will be admitted to hospital (Butler, 1980). Most of these admissions are emergencies, and in such cases children cannot be specifically prepared in advance for this experience. However, when a child's admission is planned, there is time for more specific preparation. Children and parents can be invited to visit the ward so that they can see what hospital is like. The mixture of familiar things like family groups, television and toys, with the unfamiliar and potentially frightening things like beds on wheels, outsize bathrooms, people in uniforms, and general medical equipment can be explored and explained simply and unambiguously to children. The hospital routines can be illustrated using videos or puppets, who can act out the story from admission right through to the child's return home, including parents and other close adults either visiting or staying with the child.

Children have vivid imaginations, easily fuelled by half-understood or ambiguous information which can cause them much additional fear and anxiety. It is therefore best to discuss clinical procedures and simple details of what the child will experience after admission; in language the child can easily understand. It is pointless to say that an obviously painful procedure won't hurt, and telling the child to 'be brave' will only make it harder to bear. When giving an injection the child should not be told until you have the syringe in your hand.

Facilities should be provided for either a parent or another familiar person to stay overnight with the child, and they should be encouraged to do so and shown these facilities. Where possible nurses should discuss with parents what role they should have in their child's care.

There are a number of books and games which may be useful, some of which are listed below.

For parents
Your child in hospital: a parent's handbook. Priscilla Alderson and Mary O'Toole, NAWCH. Clear and very full account of the practical side of hospital and how to work with hospital staff. Includes discussion and practical guidance on preparing your child for hospital, children's feelings about hospital, visiting, play, operations, complaints, problems.

Has your child been to hospital? Joan Woodward, NAWCH. Tells you how to cope with distressing feelings or behaviour following a stay in hospital. Describes typical feelings, fears and uncertainties of parents and children. Discusses the problem of homecoming.

For children

Going to hospital Camilla Jessel. Methuen Children's Books. 23 pages. Hardback. For pre-school children and infants. Coloured photograph on each page. The story of one child's experience. Includes weighing, measuring height, stethoscope, ear inspection, eating, oxygen mask, mother staying in, play, x-ray machines, taking medicines.

Mandy and the Hospital Alison Coles. Hodder and Stoughton. 23 Pages. Hardback. For children aged 4-10. Story of treatment following a fall. Includes tour of hospital independent of admission, outpatients, injection, toys.

Playmobil — A series of plastic figures and models. Sets include a helicopter medical unit; ambulance, doctors, nurses, patients, operating table, stretcher, and hospital beds.

Fuzzy Felt Hospital — Felt figures which can be arranged on a board to make various scenes — nurse, doctor, patients, beds and a wheelchair.

The National Association for the Welfare of Children in Hospital (NAWCH) works to raise awareness of the emotional needs of sick children and their families. NAWCH works nationally and locally to help parents before, during and after their child's stay in hospital; to persuade hospitals that parents have an essential part to play, and to publicise the needs of children in hospital in the political arena. NAWCH also undertakes research into the emotional needs of sick children, supports parents with problems, runs a library and information service, and publishes a number of books, booklets, posters, comics, slides and a Parents Pack.

For more details contact NAWCH, Argyle House, 29–31 Euston Road, London, NW1 2SD. 071-833 2041. NAWCH (Scotland), 15 Smith's Place, Edinburgh EH6 8HT. 031-553 6553. There are also local NAWCH branches throughout the United Kingdom and Ireland. Details of these can be obtained from NAWCH in London.

References

Butler, (1980) The Five Year Follow-up of the British Birth Cohort. *Health Visitor* March 1980, **53**, 81–22.

Jolly, J. (1981) The Other Side of Paediatrics, The Macmillan Press Ltd., Basingstoke.

NAWCH and Consumer's Association (1985) Children in Hospital: An action guide for parents. NAWCH, London.

Rodin, J. (1983) Will this hurt? RCN, London.

Handout: your child goes into hospital

First, some key points
You are the link between your child's everyday world and the hospital. Your child will be more confident and co-operative if you:

- Explain things in a simple and truthful way before he goes into hospital. Reassure your child that it is because you love him that you want him to get better.
- Plan to stay in the hospital if you can, otherwise be sure to visit regularly.
- Share your knowledge of your child with the hospital staff so that they can understand and help your child better.
- As far as possible, care for your child in practical ways – by feeding or washing, for example – just as you would at home.

Being prepared
It's important to talk about hospital to your children in normal conversation. Never threaten your child with a visit to hospital as a punishment. If you can, find out what facilities your local hospital has for children, so that if you need to use them you will know what to expect.

Getting ready for hospital
When you know your child is to go into hospital, explain things simply and honestly; it is very important that he can trust you completely. Playing hospital games and reading stories will help show hospitals and illness are just part of everyday life. Don't start too soon, there is a limit to what a young child can take in.

Being there
Many young children find hospitals strange and bewildering, and even more independent children need more support than usual. They need their parents with them as much as possible.

It is important for children to be with someone they love and trust, and it is DHSS policy for hospitals to make this possible – and find a bed for you when necessary – although many parents are not told about this. Be with your child as long as you and he wants, but particularly when he may be worried, eg, after going in, and before and immediately after an operation.

If possible arrange visits so that there is a familiar person nearby as often as possible, rather than have everybody arriving at once.

Long stays
If your child has a long stay in hospital or is admitted frequently, you may not be able to visit or stay as much as you would like. If you can, stay for the first few nights until the worst effects of the illness or operation are over, or until the child is used to the ward.

Working with the staff
Tell the hospital staff about any allergies to drugs or food and about any special diets and don't forget to tell them about your child's likes and dislikes. Learn how you can help. You are often welcomed to do things like washing, changing and feeding as this leaves staff free to get on with other more specialised work.

Some hospitals have interpreters for parents and children who don't speak English very well. If they don't, ask the ward sister for advice.

Leaving after visits
Many children are upset and cry when parents arrive or leave. Don't let this put you off visiting. When you leave, say goodbye calmly and leave without delay. Tell him when someone will visit next, but only if you are absolutely sure that is will be at the time you have promised.

What to pack for hospital

For your child
Favourite toy — teddy, doll or cuddly blanket, however old or scruffy
Nightwear (make sure they are marked with his name: write a list for
  the locker)
Day clothes
Sponge bag — toothbrush, toothpaste, sponge or flannel, soap, and a
  travelling soap dish
Towel
Comb, hairbrush
Dummy, bottle (even if you feel your child should have grown out of
  them — if he needs them, take them) or favourite cup
Books, small toys, games
Writing things, crayons and paper

For You
Nightwear, including dressing gown and slippers
Comfortable, cool clothes for hot wards
Watch or travel alarm
Sponge bag — toothbrush, toothpaste, sponge, soap, make-up
Towel
Change for telephone calls/drinks machine
Coffee or tea bags/thermos flask
Shampoo
Washing powder for smalls
Simple snacks eg. biscuits, cup-a-soup
Knitting, sewing or something to read
Rug and loose clothing or sleeping bag, if you have to sleep in a chair.

Help and support for parents

If you need help looking after the rest of the family because of the time you spend in hospital, ask the hospital social worker, your local social services department (look up 'Social Services' under the name of your local authority in the 'phone book), your local volunteer organiser (details from either the hospital or your local authority), or NAWCH branch if there is one.

35

Taking children at their word: pain control in paediatrics

Suzanne Alder, SRN, RSCN, DN Cert
Clinical Nurse Specialist, Great Ormond Street Hospital for Sick Children

Young children have a limited ability to understand what is happening to them and being asked of them when they are ill. Their limited experience of pain and our lack of understanding of the child's developing nervous system can only add to the obvious difficulties in measuring and, therefore, treating pain in children.

Various methods have been devised and studied to assess paediatric pain. These differ in suitability depending on the child's age, the type of pain and whether the assessment is for clinical or research purposes. Pain is subjective, so assessors must be aware of their own biases – for example culture, sex or experience, and try to remain uninfluenced by them.

Methods of assessing children's pain

Questioning   Questioning children and their parents remains one of the most common methods of pain assessment, and is useful depending on the child's age and ability to express her- or himself. The usefulness of this method can, however, be questionable.

Visual analogue scale (VAS)   Consists of a 10cm line, vertical or horizontal, with 'no pain' written at one end, and 'severe pain' at the other. Children over seven years can show how much pain they are feeling by marking this line.

Faces   Faces scales are an attempt to provide a VAS for younger children. The 'Oucher' developed by Beyer (1984) shows six expressive photographs of young children matched with a numerical scale, ranging from 0 (content) to 100 (full-blown crying). The child chooses the face which most closely approximates his or her feelings.

Poker chips   In 1979 Hester developed a numerical method in which children were given four white poker chips, and asked to select one chip if in a little pain and up to four if in great pain. This type of tool can be used successfully by children aged between four and seven years.

X marks the spot Helps children demonstrate the site of pain, although it does not quantify it. A drawing of a body outline is shown to children (aged four to 10 years) who put a cross where it hurts. A study by Eland (1977) showed that 168 of 172 children correctly placed a cross on a body outline and told the investigator why that area hurt.

Verbal scales Verbal scales such as the McGill-Melzack scale developed in 1975 are useful for adolescents who can understand adjectives such as 'lacerating' and can therefore match their pain with such a description. Younger children, however, are not able to this this so easily. Eland and Anderson (1977) describe how a six-year-old child with polio complained of his affected leg feeling like a lemon. After careful questioning, his mother established that he experienced a shrivelled-up feeling, similar to that experienced after sucking a lemon drop for a long time! It is vital to talk and listen carefully to children and establish exactly what they mean.

Pain diary These can be helpful especially to record the pattern of chronic pain, avoiding the discrepancy between reports by children and their parents, and to assess the effects of treatment prescribed.

Some people choose to measure children's pain by observing their behaviour. This can be successful, but difficulties arise distinguishing between pain and other forms of distress, defining 'normal' behaviour and observing children accurately and consistently. Formal behaviour charts are sometimes used in research, although for a young baby or child drowsy following general anaesthetic, informal observation may be the only method available of assessing pain.

Crying is the usual way parents or healthcare professionals assess whether a baby or child is in pain. Wolff (1969) described how the pain cry differs from a hunger cry, but in real life this is not always so clear.

Other forms of behaviour associated with pain in babies and children include change of facial expression, body rigidity and movement of the affected part. Even if young children can demonstrate the presence of pain by such behavioural changes, it must be remembered a child suffering from chronic pain may be able to 'mute out' behavioural responses even when still in pain.

Although observing physiological changes in both children and adults has been used widely as a method of pain assessment (blood pressure, pulse, respiration rate, sweating and hormonal changes), this has rarely proved useful in children, as these signs are influenced by too many variables, such as fear, stress or the illness itself. They have, however, proved useful in babies. Williamson and Williamson (1983) showed infants who received a penile block for circumcision had lower heart rates than those who received no anaesthetic block. Anand *et al* (1985) used these techniques to condemn the practice of ligating patent ductus arterioses in babies with inadequate analgesia.

Pain is made up of physiological, psychological, social, ethnic and cultural components. In most situations more than one of these contributes to what the child feels, while staff attitudes to assessment and treatment also affect the child. Fear and anxiety contribute towards pain, and in hospitalised children feared or actual separation from their parents can add to the fear of medical procedures.

Previous pain experience and parental influence are significant factors in the amount of pain felt by children. After the age of six months, for example, a child will remember certain aspects of an injection procedure such as the needle, a white coat, or being restrained, and might act fearfully if required to repeat the experience. Adolescents whose parents are over-protective or over-involved in their child's activities, seem less able to cope with pain than those whose parents are not as intrusive.

Different cultures respond to pain in different ways: Italians, for example, believe it is natural to cry and moan when in pain and therefore are seen as having a low pain tolerance. Children naturally follow their parents' reactions – in our society it is commonly accepted that 'men don't cry', and therefore adolescent boys experiencing pain may try to hide their suffering, as they feel they are expected to be brave. Even young children can be affected by these beliefs. Eland and Anderson (1977) describe how a six-year-old boy who received multiple injuries after being struck by a car denied feeling any pain when asked in the presence of his father. The child was interviewed the following day, this time when his aunt was in the room. When asked about pain he burst into tears – he was able to say in front of his aunt that he was in pain and had been on many occasions since the accident.

Nurses' own fears influence pain management. Many believe that by giving an unwilling child an injection, for example, they will come into disfavour with the child. Some nurses are so worried about being seen as a 'baddie' that their fears actually stop them giving a much needed injection to a child in pain.

Nurses and other healthcare professionals can also make subjective judgements about the pain level a child is experiencing, regarding a child as a 'sissy' or having a low pain threshold if he or she complains. "Children do not experience pain with the intensity that adults do" and "Narcotics always depress respiration in children" are opinions voiced on and off the ward. It is not surprising therefore, that children are sometimes left to suffer from untreated pain.

Acute pain

Peri/postoperative pain   A common cause of pain in children, this is now more readily acknowledged. However, until recently there has been "traditional reluctance to prescribe analgesic drugs to alleviate postoperative or other pain" in neonates and young children, due to doubts as to whether neonates feel pain and concerns over potentially harmful effects of powerful analgesics, such as respiratory depression or even addiction (Hatch, 1987). Anyone who has witnessed the restraint needed for a newborn undergoing a simple operative procedure such as circumcision without general anaesthetic, will have little doubt of a neonate's ability to feel pain (Eland and Anderson, 1977). Patient controlled analgesia is a method of postoperative pain control used with adults, which is beginning to be explored in paediatrics.

Medical interventions   All children are subjected to pain from medical procedures at some time during their lives, such as heel pricks when tiny babies, or immunisations. There is evidence that children who are subjected to frequent interventions become sensitised to these procedures, and their fears become greater each time they visit the hospital. Doctors and nurses, however, frequently ignore this aspect of pain, with comments like "it will only take a few seconds" or "are we going to be brave today?"

Accidents and injuries   Accidents are the biggest cause of death in children, and accidental injury is one of the biggest causes of childhood pain. Accidents such as car crashes, falls, burns and scalds, cuts and lacerations are extremely common.

Chronic pain

Juvenile chronic arthritis   Passo (1982) found that 4.5 per cent of children have sufficient pain to interfere with their daily activities for more than three months. Juvenile chronic arthritis can seriously debilitate children and cause extended periods of pain and suffering.

Abdominal pain   Caused by a variety of disorders, recurrent abdominal pain can occur with no detectable organic cause. This problem is quite common, affecting 12.3 per cent of girls and 9.5 per cent of boys (Apley and Naish, 1958). If no organic cause is found, it should not simply be assumed that the pain is psychogenic.

Headache   Most of us suffer from headaches at some stage in our lives. Despite the multiple obvious causes of headache, there are some children who suffer ongoing headaches for no apparent reason.

Cancer   Most children suffering from cancer suffer pain at some stage. The psychological effects and implications can often increase this pain dramatically, especially if they are not attended to sympathetically. It can be difficult – sometimes impossible – to untangle the physical pain felt by the child from the psychological pain caused by fear, watching distraught parents and worrying about the outcome of the disease.

Treatment of pain

There are many treatments for children's pain and those chosen will depend on the assessment of the pain and its cause. It is important to remain objective when planning treatment, but the causes of pain and any relevant social and cultural factors must be taken into account.

Numerous analgesics are available and it helps to remember a few important points. The correct strength analgesia should be given to correspond with the amount of pain the child is suffering. The 'analgesic' ladder is important to remember when prescribing drugs for children, as if the chosen drug is too mild it will not have the desired effect and the child may refuse further pain relief. If the drug is too strong, or the dose too high, it will have adverse effects on the child. It is better to know a few drugs well than to have a poor understanding of a wide range.

In chronic pain, always give analgesia regularly so the child is not experiencing peaks and troughs in pain control. Mild analgesics such as paracetamol and aspirin can be effective, especially if given regularly (every four to six hours), and dosage depends on the child's age and weight. It often surprises people that in the control of chronic pain from cancer, mild analgesics will often keep the child pain free for several weeks before a stronger drug is required.

The next rung on the ladder are mild opioids such as Dihydrocodeine and codeine which should be given on a regular basis, with dose depending on the age and weight of the child.

If the mild opioids are no longer effective, the next and final step are strong opioids such as morphine and diamorphine. Again, these must be given regularly to ensure adequate pain relief. Morphine sulphate slow release tablets (MST), have a long half life and therefore only need to be given every 12 hours. This can obviously be helpful to parents, who may have previously been battling with their child every four hours to encourage him or her to take medication. The starting dose for MST is 1mg/kg twice daily. Pain caused by nerve compression can be difficult to manage, and is not usually responsive to opioid drugs. Tricyclic antidepressant drugs such as amitriptyline may be helpful. Also anti-epileptic drugs such as carbomazepine may be helpful for neuropathic pain.

Routes of administration
Once an analgesic has been selected, an appropriate route of administration must be chosen. The oral route is first choice, but unfortunately is not always as easy as it sounds – we've all tried administering medicine to a toddler, ending up with most of it in our laps! Even though many modern medicines are pleasant tasting, trying to persuade children to take them can be extremely difficult. Parental involvement, the use of play including dolls and teddies being given medicine first, disguising tablets with sugar and jam, and nurses' patience and attitudes are all important.

When a child cannot take oral medication, another route must be chosen. Intramuscular codeine phosphate is often the drug of choice for babies postoperatively, especially when they are breathing spontaneously and strong opioids are being avoided, whereas intramuscular omnopon is often prescribed for bigger children.

Infusion if a more effective way of administering postoperative analgesia, however, giving the child constant pain relief rather than peaks and troughs. Diamorphine is sometimes given at doses of 0.5mg/kg over one to two days. Postoperative epidural analgesia is extremely effective but depends on nurses being trained to look after the infusion and is not always practical in a busy surgical environment.

In terminally ill children who can no longer tolerate oral medication, subcutaneous diamorphine is effective. This is given via a syringe pump, which is easy to use and fairly inexpensive, so parents, or even the children, can often learn to operate it. The small size of the machine allows children to remain active for as long as their condition allows.

Intravenous diamorphine can also be given continuously via a syringe driver, but there is no advantage over the subcutaneous route. However, if a long line such as a Hickman line is *in situ*, this will avoid inflicting more needles upon the child. Rectal morphine is also available for children for whom other routes are not appropriate, but steady pain control can be difficult to achieve, probably due to absorption problems.

Problems with morphine and diamorphine

Although opioids are extremely effective in relieving pain in children, their use will always incur some anxiety. Parents sometimes become worried at the thought of their child using opioids, fearing he or she might become hooked on drugs. It is, therefore, important to prepare parents who may also worry about physical changes and respiratory problems – showing them pictures of other children on similar drugs, and who still look the same and are continuing with their normal lives will help.

Unfortunately, many professionals still believe some of the myths about morphine and diamorphine, denying analgesia to children in intense pain (Eland and Anderson, 1977). A study of adults and children with identical diagnoses matched only 18 of the 25 children by diagnosis. The 18 adults received 372 narcotic analgesics and 299 non-narcotics – a total of 671 doses, while the 25 children received a total of 24 doses of analgesics. Although incidences of respiratory depression have occurred in neonates, probably because of altered pharmacokinetics and increased sensitivity to opioids related to the blood brain barrier, safe use of opioids in children is possible providing the correct dose is given. If respiratory depression does occur, it can be reversed by giving Naloxone.

Reluctance to use these drugs must be weighed up against the often troublesome side effects of reduced movement and the humane aspect of human suffering. Fears of addiction also prevent some doctors from prescribing opioids to children, but if the correct dose is given and this is titrated as the child recovers, dependence is easily controlled. There are few side effects, but they affect most children to a greater or lesser degree (Table 1). However, the benefits usually outweigh the side effects in most parents' minds.

Drowsiness Quite a common effect in the first few days, but almost always wears off once the child is accustomed to the drug.
Constipation Common with all forms of opioid analgesia, if constipation is recognised early, or better still, prevented by giving a laxative regularly, it can be controlled.
Nausea and vomiting These are uncommon in children, and can usually be controlled with the use of appropriate anti-emetics and careful diet. May be due to an incorrect dosage.
Hallucinations and nightmares These problems occur occasionally when a child is commenced on opioids, and usually wear off within 48 hours.
Itching This can be quite a problem to some children. It usually wears off when the child is accustomed to the drug, but may be eased by topical or systemic antihistamines or calamine lotion.

Table 1. Side effects of opioid drugs.

Psychological methods of pain relief

Fear can add to the painful experience of being ill and is a problem which should be tackled actively and sympathetically. Many hospitals now produce pamphlets and books for young children to see before a planned hospital admission, and parents are encouraged to stay with their children in hospital, participating as much as possible in their care. Brothers and sisters are also encouraged to visit, and in Nottingham, even pets are encouraged on to the children's unit (Ainsworth, 1989).

Allowing a terminally ill child and his or her family the choice to go home, providing adequate support is available, is of the utmost importance. Most families, given this choice, will wish to take their child home, and a dying child can then spend the last days away from the stresses of hospital life, in the comfort and security of home.

Full explanations and constant reassurance are vital to keep children as relaxed as possible and maintain their trust. Children often believe pain is a punishment for having done wrong, and all sorts of ideas and fantasies may fill their minds if they are not kept informed of what is happening to them and why.

Hypnosis has been found to be successful in dealing with children's pain in many cases. Particular problems such as needle phobia and pain during medical procedures can be helped using this method.

Distraction techniques and the use of imagery and relaxation methods are similarly helpful, especially if parents join in too. These require relatively little time to learn, are cheap and unobtrusive and allow older children to gain some control over their fears. These techniques are demonstrated in a Canadian video 'No Fears, No Tears'.

Local methods of pain control

There are various other methods to reduce pain, which can be valuable alongside other forms of analgesia:

EMLA (enteric mixture of local anaesthetics) is a local anaesthetic cream which prevents pain during venepuncture. It should be applied to the chosen area one hour before the procedure and covered with an occlusive dressing. This cream helps many children overcome their fear of needles.

Skin coolant sprays can also be used before childhood immunisations, while topical heat, in the form of heat pads, and cold such as ice packs, are useful for complaints such as abdominal pain or bruising.

The use of transcutaneous electrical nerve stimulation (TENS) can be helpful for phantom limb pain, postoperative pain, and even pain from more serious conditions such as deaferentation pain from cancer.

Radiotherapy is a painless procedure which can be used particularly for children with localised pain from cancer, and is very useful for dying children, whose quality of life can often be improved for days or even weeks, by a short course of radiotherapy to a problem area. Entonox (nitrous oxide and oxygen) has proved effective and safe in children of four years and over. It is self-administered via a mask or mouthpiece, and can be used during short procedures such as suturing, plastering, removing sutures and changing dressings.

Homoeopathic remedies and acupuncture are chosen by some parents for their children – indeed may be the first choice of treatment in some instances. We must remember that freedom of choice is everyone's perogative, and even if our beliefs differ we are not necessarily right.

Pain suffered by young children can be reduced by a wide variety of remedies. Each child will feel pain of differing levels and degrees, and react to, and cope with this in their own way. As healthcare professionals, we have an obligation to children suffering from pain – the choice of pain relief methods and the tools available to measure and assess pain mean there is little excuse or reason for any child to suffer. The lack of research, at least until recently, into paediatric pain, means more exploration and assessment are required to help us tackle the problem effectively. We have a duty to dispel some of the old myths about paediatric pain.

References

Ainsworth, H. (1989) And the guinea pig came too. *Nursing Times,* **85,** 39, 55–56.

Anand, K.J.S. and Aynsley-Green, A. (1985) Metabolic and endocrine effects of surgical ligation of patent ductus arteriosus in the human preterm neonate: Are there implications for further improvement of postoperative outcome? Mod. Pr *Paediatrics,* 23, 143–157.

Apley, J. and Naish, N. (1958). Children with recurrent abdominal pains; a field survey of 1,000 School Children. *Archives of Disease in Childhood,* **33,** 165–170.

Beyer, J.E. (1984) *The Oucher: a user's manual and technical report.* The Hospital Play Equipment Co., Evanston, Il.

Eland, J.M. (1977). *Children's Experience of Pain: A Descriptive Study.* Unpublished data.

Eland, J.M. and Anderson, J.E. (1977) *Pain.* Little Brown & Co, Boston.

Goldman, A. and Lloyd-Thomas, A.R. (in press). Management of pain in children and neonates. British Medical Bulletin, **47,** (3).

Hatch, D.J. (1987) Analgesia in the neonate. *BMJ,* **294,** 6577, 920.

McGrath, P.J. and Unruh, A.M. (1989) *Pain in Children and Adolescents.* Elsener, pp 73–104.

Melzack, R. (1975) The McGill-Melzack Pain Questionnaire: major properties and scoring methods. *Pain,* **1,** 277-99.

Passo, M.H. (1982). Aches and limb pain. *Paediatr. Clin. North Am,* **29,** 209-19.

Williamson, P.S. and Williamson, M.L. (1983). Physiologic stress reduction by a local anaesthetic during newborn circumcision. *Paediatrics,* 71, 36-40.

Wolff, P.H. (1969) The natural history of crying and other vocalisations in early infancy. In: B.M. Foss (Ed). *Determinants of Infant Behaviour,* Vol 4, Methuen, London.

36

Communicating with children

June Jolly, SRN, RSCN
Child Health Co-ordinator, Greenwich Health Authority

'Well, what's so different about that?'; 'I find them rather intimidating, don't you?'; 'They either ask impossible questions or start howling when you've only tried to explain what you are going to do.'; 'I don't know either, I can never get a sensible answer to the most elementary of questions.'

Such comments show why communicating with children must be taken seriously. Children's reasoning powers are commensurate with their mental and, frequently, physical age. Their understanding is limited not only by their vocabulary but also their life experience. The child who has grown up in the inner city will be more likely to be familiar with tubes and escalators – but try explaining what they are to an immigrant child, or one from the provinces of a very sheltered or deprived environment. When it comes to the child who needs hospital care, as a casualty, an out or in-patient, the task becomes more formidable. It is unlikely that anything will be familiar and the very strangeness of the environment added to pain or bewilderment will make it even more difficult to understand. The best way is to explain the parent who can then interpret to the child. This, of course, is not always possible. Then a knowledge of the developmental processes which govern the child's increasing understanding and logical reasoning power will help.

For example – at six to seven months the baby recognises and shows fear of strangers. Aged one to three the toddler learns the meaning of 'No' and the power of using it and also becomes adventurous but has no sense of danger. Children under four rarely understand the concept of 'tomorrow' and, emotionally, relationships will be as they are to a mother. To 'go away' may imply 'never come back'. Most children suffer form separation anxiety throughout the pre-school years, if parted from their parents.

Children under six are not always aware of their bodies as an integral part of themselves. But is is then they start to view an assault of one part as a threat to their whole being. Development of moral judgement and adult logical reasoning will not be complete until 10 to 12 years. It may still be confusing because the child has his own way of reasoning, and to slot into this may be the most helpful.

Real-life situations

The following are real-life situations which could form the basis of discussion between yourself and colleagues.

Situation 1 Tim and Jenny had been admitted to their local hospital for tonsillectomy and were taken to the children's ward. The nurse told them about what would happen. She asked whether they knew where their tonsils were? Both pointed to their throats. She got them both to peer into each other's throats to see where they were. By putting out their tongues and panting like puppies they had a good view, and it was fun, too. She then explained about the magic sleep the doctor would give them and the special magic cream that would make sure they wouldn't feel anything – all very good. Asked how the doctor would get the tonsils out, Tim became very dubious. Using his index finger he took a quick slice across his throat from ear to ear and at the same time made a grimace. Jenny was horrified. Both children were between four and five.

How could the nurse reassure them that this barbaric procedure was not what would happen?

(a) Give a simple straightforward explanation of the way the surgeon operated.

(b) Use language and vocabulary with which the children were familiar to explain how their mouths could be opened whilst they were asleep.

(c) Merely promise them they would be asleep and wouldn't feel anything.

Obviously the children would need explanation in terms they would understand. They also needed reassurance that they wouldn't be awake of feel anything. Sometimes in trying to be truthful we go into too much detail. Look at children's stories. They go into detail about very little, and then it is usually over the trivial or smaller issues. There is no need to give explanation about a procedure, but it is important to explain the things that worry the child.

Will they be sure to be asleep? How could they open their mouths – and would they stay open? How does the doctor get at the tonsils?

It is better to avoid using terms like scalpels, forceps, which they don't understand, or even knives or razors with which they might start experimenting later on their friends. A good plan is to describe events that the child will consciously remember. What he does not know will not normally matter to him. He will ask for information he wants. You do not need to do more than answer what he asks.

Situation 2 Philip aged six had orthopaedic surgery for correction of a congenital malformation of his leg, requiring a plaster cast. He was an only child of articulate parents who explained that the doctor would mend his leg so that he could play football like Daddy. He helped pack his nightclothes and chose some toys and games to take with him. His mother promised she would sleep there too and he was quite excited. In the ward the nurse showed him his bed and locker and introduced him to other children. He was told about the operation but it was not the custom to go into details of the surgery or to 'practise' wearing operation gowns etc. After surgery he appeared to make a good recovery. Next day however this usually chatty West Indian boy was silent. Even his parents could not get him to speak and he remained withdrawn for several weeks, making them feel he was blaming them and couldn't trust them anymore.

What clues are there to help 'get inside his mind' to see what the trouble was ?

(a) Why might Philip have felt he was being punished? What sort of things do parents say inadvertently?

(b) Had he been let down by this hospitalisation?
    What might his family have neglected to tell him?

(c) Had the plaster of paris on his leg been what he had expected and what did it mean?

(a) and (b) It is unlikely that having been prepared by his mother and the hospital staff that he really felt he was being 'punished'. The fact that his mother stayed with him should have alleviated any anxiety that this had happened because he wasn't loved.

(b) Children of this age do not always understand things in an adult fashion. Whereas an adult may wonder how a hard plaster of paris could be removed, children may assume it is a permanent alternative limb. If this was compounded by the shock of finding it white, he could well have been shocked. A good way of teaching children about plaster of paris casts is to let them help put a small one on a favourite doll or model. By cutting it off with scissors after it had hardened, gives a child much more confidence that this could and will happen, than any amount of explaining.

Situation 3   Julie aged seven had been in hospital for a few days with a severe infection for which she needed antibiotics. On the third day she objected strongly to the injection so the nurse said "don't worry, I'll give it by mouth instead". The child became hysterical. Why? She misinterpreted the nurse and thought she would be given the injection into her mouth. How could the nurse have made sure she understood and was reassured?

(a) Explained that the alternative way of giving the medicine was in a syrup which she could swallow.

(b) Shown her the medicine and the measure or spoon. Discuss other ways in which the child might have been reassured and not terrified.

This is a good example of a child's 'defective' understanding. No adult would have imagined that an injection would be given into the mouth. By mouth is well understood by adults. But why should children have this knowledge? There are many illustrations that could be given for this sort of misunderstanding. Any explaining. Any explanation needs to be carefully worded and preferably accompanied by a visual aid, either on yourself, another adult (Mummy for preference) or a doll.

Situation 4 Barry, aged five, had been diagnosed as having a defect in his heart. His family had an open and positive attitude towards Barry's difficulty. One day he asked his mother – 'Will I be able to love when I grow up?'.

His mother asked him, 'Why do you think you won't be able to love?' to which he replied, 'Well I've got something wrong with my heart so I thought I couldn't.'

How would you have answered his question? Do you think that would have elicited the reply the mother got?

The principle of reflecting a question is even more valid with children than with adults. When a child asks what appears to be a 'stupid' or obtuse question it is worth finding out what he really means before coming in with a trite answer.

Situation 5 The words in the box are taken at randon from the ward furniture. Among yourselves try to explain what each item is so that a child would understand its use.

Bed table	Suction machine	Monkey pole
Traction	Suction catheter	Patella hammer
Oxygen tent	Incubator	Bedpan/bottle
Bed cradle	Syringe driver	Operation gown

Now look at the words again and try to imagine what a child might think you meant when hearing you use it initially. This will give you a good insight into how children can so easily get the 'wrong end of the stick.'

Bibliography
Donaldson, M. (1978) *Children's Minds.* Fontana/Collins, London. A new approach to Piaget's theory of development.
Jolly, J. (1981) *The Other Side of Paediatrics.* Macmillan Education, Basingstoke. Meeting the every day needs of children who have to be in hospital.
McLeod Clark, J. and Bridge, W. (1981) *Communication in Nursing Care.* HM&M, Aylesbury. Includes a chapter on communication
Petrillo M. and Sangers, S. (1980) *Emotional Care of Hospitalised children.* Lippincot, Philadelphia. Definitive work on communicating with children and meeting their emotional needs.
Rodin, J. (1983) *Does it hurt?* RCN Monograph. Research on children's concepts of hospital and medical tests and their need to be prepared.

37

Parents in the anaesthetic room: a blessing or a curse?

Alan Glasper, BA, RGN, RSCN, ONC, DN, Cert Ed, RNT
Professor of Nursing, University of Southampton

The presence of parents in the anaesthetic room has received scant attention in nursing, medical or psychology literature, especially in the UK. However, Hanallah (1983), Schulman (1967) and Merrick (1983) have studied the effects of parental presence during anaesthesia and all are favourably disposed. Schulman's study concentrated on 32 children admitted for tonsillectomy. The group accompanied by a parent proved to be less upset than the unaccompanied group. Schulman agreed that upset during induction was mitigated by the mother's presence. It is interesting to note that no mothers turned down the invitation to accompany their children and all were cooperative and enthusiastic about the experience.

In Hanallah's study the parents of 50 unpremedicated children were invited to be present during the induction of anaesthesia. The mood of each child was assessed at four stages:

- the waiting room;

- the preinductive period;

- during induction;

- postoperatively in the recovery room.

Hanallah concluded that for some preschool children parental presence

---

Factors operating against parental accompaniment

1. Local custom — operating department rules and regulations.
2. Fear of increased risk of infection.
3. Potential problems of coping with two potential patients — parents may require attention, especially if they faint.
4. Training expriences may be hampered by parental presence.
5. Fear of having a potential critic in the anaesthetic room.

during the induction of anaesthesia proved effective in relieving anxiety and in reducing the need for premedication.

Merrick's study looked at the significance of parental presence and showed that the anaesthetic staff found it helpful in 31 cases, immaterial in seven cases, a little harmful in one case and very harmful in a further case.

Changes

The Platt Report in 1959 recommended sweeping changes in the way children were cared for in hospital. It advocated unrestricted visiting and the desirability of providing residential accommodation for parents, particularly those of children below school age, but its findings were largely ignored by many paediatric units. The absence of radical change proved to be the precursor for the formation of the National Association for the Welfare of Children in Hospital (NAWCH) in 1961. Some 26 years later the original objective of NAWCH to implement the recommendations of Platt on a national basis has still to be achieved in some paediatric units.

In 1976 the Court Report highlighted further inadequacies in the way children were cared for in hospital. In particular it called for pressing improvements in the training of staff and exhorted institutions to devote greater resources for the special needs of children. Much remains to be done before it can be said that the joint philosophies of Platt and Court have been fulfilled. However, the move towards unrestricted visiting, parental accommodation and now care-by-parent units has ensured a growing trend towards family centred care.

Psychological upset

It has been demonstrated that some children may benefit from a hospital experience (Vernon and Schulman, 1964) but preschool children are especially vulnerable, old enough to suffer the stresses and yet too young to profit fully from any psychological preparation that may be available. Separation from parents is a major cause of psychological upset in preschool children both immediate and long term, but can be mitigated by reducing parental separation. Although the role of parents has increased in recent years, for various reasons parents have not taken, or have not been allowed to take, full advantage of what appears to be new opportunities to become involved in the care of their child during a hospital stay. Such opportunities are being reflected in the gradual introduction of preadmission programmes and care-by-parent schemes to UK paediatric units. Although at an early stage of development, such innovations are gradually highlighting the natural resource that paediatric nurses have at their disposal in the form of parents and guardians. The parent, as an equal partner in the traditional nurse/doctor/patient relationship, should accelerate this change.

R.M. Smith (1968) has stated: ''In children (who are) old enough to have fear or apprehension (during surgery) the emotional factor may be an even greater source of concern than the child's physical condition. (It is often) in fact the greater problem of the entire operative course.'' In order to avoid separation completely and thereby reduce upset, some anaesthetic departments allow parents to accompany their children to the anaesthetic room and remain with them until they are asleep. Some anaesthetists go one step further and allow parental presence in the recovery room.

J. Ross Mackenzie (1927) stated that: ''The mental condition of the patient may be highly detrimental to the safe induction and maintenance of anaesthesia.'' Here, of course, Mackenzie was principally referring to adults, thus demonstrating that people of all ages have a dread of anaesthesia, arising perhaps from the subconscious fear that they may not wake up, or that the surgeon may begin the operation before they are fully anaesthetised. This fear has long been recognised and the use of heavy premedicants ensured, at least for many patients, that they were asleep before they ever arrived in the anaesthetic room. Sleep induction (ie the use of sedative premedicants) was widely used in paediatrics and in many ways prevented the types of anxiety seen today. The gradual decline of sedative premedicants is, ironically, linked with the changing patterns of management of sick children. To reduce separation and the effects of hospitalisation, there has been a growing demand for day surgery — where the child is admitted in the morning and discharged in the afternoon. This practice, laudable though it is, has prevented many anaesthetists using sleep induction and has ensured that most children are awake when they arrive in the anaesthetic room.

Children's perception

The mind of the preschool, preoperational child is unable to comprehend such concepts of reversibility and many children appear to experience the impending anaesthetic as a death threat (Balberie, 1985). Telling a child he is going to be put to sleep is hardly reassuring when one considers what happens to pets when they are put to sleep.

The trip to the anaesthetic room can, in itself, be a daunting experience for a child. Long corridors, lifts and strange faces often wearing masks all combine to cause fear and apprehension in a child who, less than an hour earlier, had been in his own home. For many day-case children it is the final straw in a day that began without breakfast or even a drink, a day when, after arriving in a strange building and having a strange man examine him (even though mummy has repeatedly asked him not to talk to strangers) he had a painful injection in the leg by a strange lady in a funny dress.

The author is currently investigating the effect of parental presence during the induction of anaesthesia and hypothesises that children are less upset when accompanied by their parents. Behaviour differences between accompanied and unaccompanied children are being studied, using video tape.

Questionnaire

An article in the *British Medical Journal* (White, 1985) advocating the accompaniment of children to the anaesthetic room by parents caused a flurry of correspondence among interested parties. Many contrasting views were expressed. Following the publication of these letters a postal questionnaire (Glasper and Dewar, 1986) was sent to all 67 members of the Association of British Paediatric Anaesthetists. It was deemed appropriate to approach anaesthetists as only they have the final say as to whether parents accompany their children to the anaesthetic room. Obviously this group represents only a small proportion of the number of anaesthetists who deliver anaesthetics to children and yet it was hoped to obtain a 'weather gauge' of the practices regarding parental presence around the UK. Of the 67 questionnaires posted, 35 responses (52 per cent) were received. The results of this simple questionnaire were as predicted and validated the available literature on the subject.

The aim of the postal questionnaire was to ascertain the views and opinions regarding parental presence and to highlight areas of agreement and disagreement among members of the association. The questionnaire addressed three main areas:

- policies relating to parental presence;

- practices regarding the use of premedication;

- attitudes and opinions relating to parental presence.

Policy Twelve respondents had written policies regarding parental presence at the induction of anaesthesia, and 18 gave parents the choice of accompanying their children to the anaesthetic room and remaining with them during induction. Where parental presence at the induction of anaesthesia was accepted, 26 respondents allowed one parent only, with three respondents allowing both. Where a policy on parental presence existed, its implementation in 12 out of 14 cases was at the discretion of the anaesthetist. The responsibility of the anaesthetist is to the patient and during the particularly stressful period of induction some anaesthetists worry that they may have an extra patient in the form of a parent, especially as some may faint.

Where parents accompany their children to the anaesthetic room the majority of respondents indicated that some form of protective clothing is worn, often in a variety of combinations ranging from overclothes to complete changes of clothing. In four areas parents were also asked to wear masks. This is particularly interesting as only one respondent agreed that the presence of parents in the anaesthetic room represented an infection hazard.

Practices regarding the use of premedication When asked if premedication is generally unnecessary when children are accompanied to the anaesthetic room by a parent, only six anaesthetists agreed. Johnson and Young's study (1986) indicated that placebo was considerably more effective as a premedicant than was Trimeprazine. The use of atropine in very young children is undeniably essential due to the relatively small size of their airways. The optimum method of administration remains unclear and there are still many paediatric units who favour the intramuscular route. The rapid utilisation of topical local anaesthetic creams to facilitate painless intravenous inductions throughout UK paediatric units belies the negative response appertaining to the use of such creams when the survey was conducted early in 1986.

Attitudes and opinions related to parental presence   When asked if parents should accompany their children to the anaesthetic room and remain with them during the induction of anaesthesia whenever possible, 17 respondents agreed or strongly agreed. Sixteen agreed that children are less anxious during the induction of anaesthesia when accompanied by a parent, 12 respondents agreed that the induction of anaesthesia where parents are present is generally easier and 14 respondents agreed that parental presence should be encouraged in the recovery areas.

The results confirmed there is a dichotomy of opinion relating to the subject and, in view of the paucity of UK data, the central problem must be to study benefits and problems associated with parental presence.

- Does parental presence contribute to the welfare of the children?

- Does parental presence cause further problems?

- Does parental presence cause unacceptable problems for anaesthetists, surgeons and nursing staff?

- Does parental presence increase the risk of infection?

The wide variety of opinion and practice related to the subject suggests that some investigation may unmask the confusion.

References

Balberie, R. (1985) Fear is the key. *Senior Nurse*, **3**, 4.

Court, (1976) *Fit for the Future: Report of the Court Committee*, HMSO, London.

Glasper, E.A. and Dewar, A. (1986) The results of a postal questionnaire appertaining to parental presence at the induction of anaesthesia. Unpublished.

Hanallah, R.S. *et al* (1983) Experience with parents' presence during anaesthesia induction in children. *Canadian Anaesthesia Society Journal*, **30**, 3, 386_389.

Johnson, T.W. and Young, P.M. (1986) Premedication for children. *Anaesthesia*, **41**.

Mackenzie, J.R. (1927) A lecture on anaesthetics, *The Lancet*, Jan. 22.

Merrick, J. *et al*   (1983) The presence of parents at out-patient operations on children. *Ugeskr Laeger*, **145**, 3041–4.

Platt Report (1989) The Welfare of Children in Hospital: Report of the Platt Committee. HMSO, London.

Schulman, J.L. *et al* (1967) A study of the effect of the mother's presence during anaesthesia induction. *Paediatrics*, **39**, 1.

Smith, R.M. (1968) Anaesthesia for Infants and Children. (3rd Ed.) Mosby, St. Louis.

Vernon, D.T.A. and Schulman, J.L. (1964) Hospitalisation as a source of psychological benefit to children. *Paediatrics*, **36**, 11, 694–696.

While, J. *et al* (1985) Personal view. *British Medical Journal*, **291**, 343.

Bibliography

Hain, W. (1980) Children in hospital. *Anaesthesia*, **35**, 949–951.

This article discusses the role of parents in the anaesthetic room.

Quinton, D., Rutter, M. (1976) Early hospital admissions and later disturbances of behaviour. *Develop. Med. Child Neurol*, **18**.

A general article on stress in children admitted to hospital.

38

Caring by parents

Margaret Evans, RGN, RSCN, BSc (Hons) in Nursing Studies
Nurse Specialist in Paediatric Oncology, Southampton University Hospital

Welfare of children in hospital

The welfare of children in hospital has been brought into focus by several writers, the most notable of these being John Bowlby who commented on the importance of attachment. Bowlby (1953) felt that healthy social development depended upon attachment to a consistent 'mother figure' and that separation could result in later maladjustment.

James Robertson's book *Young Children in Hospital* (1958) supported Bowlby's theories and provided a scientific basis for the admission of families to hospitals with their children. This work influenced the findings of the Platt Report (1959) as did the work of Bowlby. This report, *The Welfare of Children in Hospital*, was the first DHSS report specifically concerned with the needs of children in hospital. It heralded much needed change in paediatric care, which had been mostly based on an inappropriate adult model of care. Up until that time little provision had been made for the very different needs of children, restricted visiting being the most outstanding example.

Platt recommended that:

- children be nursed in appropriate units.
- children be cared for by qualified paediatric nurses.
- families should be involved as much as possible in all aspects of care and in all decisions.
- there should be unrestricted visiting together with accommodation for parents.
- play and educational facilities should be available.
- children should be discharged into the community as soon as possible.

In 1961, the National Association for the Welfare of Children in Hospital (NAWCH) was founded, its aim being to encourage the implementation of the Platt Report. NAWCH, being a successful pressure group, have produced several reports concerned with various aspects of child welfare in hospital.

Continuing concern was expressed in the Court Report (1976) which emphasised the importance of family centred care for children. In August 1988, the DHSS/DOH mounted a major review of services for children in hospital and comprehensive guidelines on the welfare of children in hospital have now been produced (DHSS, 1990).

It is clear, then, that although there are pockets of resistance, paediatric nursing has made major advances over the last thirty years. This has been stimulated by various reports, as well as by research and much anecdotal evidence which has consistently shown that unsupported hospitalization can cause long-term behavioural problems in children. Providing a suitable environment with adequate play and educational facilities must alleviate some of the child's anguish, but it is quite clear that the root cause of the disturbance is separation from the 'mother figure'.

Role of parents It is therefore strongly suggested that a parent's presence in hospital makes a major contribution to a child's welfare. Parents have a unique body of knowledge regarding their child and are able to provide security, continuity and support. They are also well able to perform much of the nursing care for their child. As early as 1947, Spence strongly supported this view when he discussed the care of children in hospital in the British Medical Journal. He recommended that care by parent units should be instituted because by far the greatest part of sick children's nursing is already done by mothers in their homes.

Since 1947, of course, parental involvement in care has evolved (albeit slowly) to satisfy the child's psychosocial upheaval and the parent's need to retain a degree of control over a stressful situation. It may also have evolved due to low staffing levels, where parents find themselves supplementing nursing care, and it is clear that the parents' role could be abused in this situation.

The 1980s have certainly been characterised by the paediatric nurse accepting the many advantages of being involved in a partnership with parents and as Webb (1985) noted most parents are keen to do more than nursing staff think they are capable of doing.

Care by parents

Glasper (1990) observed that although the underlying concept of care by patients originated in the UK, it was in North America that it actually took root. Although Spence advocated the idea in 1947, there are only two documented research pieces on the subject in the UK (Sainsbury *et al*, 1986; Evans, 1990). Many centres in the UK are certainly pursuing the idea, notably Nottingham (Fradd, 1988), The Hospital for Sick Children, London (Casey, 1988) and the Royal Marsden Hospital. In the US several research projects and several papers have been published and the concept appears to be well established in many centres.

Definition of care by parents

Oberlander (1983) describes what developed in a care by parent unit in America over a fourteen year period. She saw it as being one where no physical care need be provided by the nurses, because in most cases responsible parents were capable of delivering that care. She saw the nurse, however, as being there to provide education and support, and being in a position to take over from parents, when necessary.

Evans *et al* (1983) discuss the therapeutic advantages of parental involvement, arguing that it can take various forms from the parent being seated by the bedside, to assuming some degree of caring responsibility, to care by parent rooms where parents nurse their children under the supervision of the nursing staff.

Sainsbury (1986) portrays the concept succinctly when he describes the care by parent system as one which clarifies the role of the parents and gives them an active participation and responsibility in the healing process.

Most recent writers on the subject now argue for the parent being involved in as much of the child's care as is possible for that individual parent.

Advantages of care by parents

It would be realistic to say that most paediatric units recommend the continuous presence of a parent while a child is in hospital, and in paediatric practice any philosophy which negates this is unacceptable. It is, therefore, not necessary to discuss the advantage of a parental presence in hospital, but rather to discuss the advantage of parents actually being involved in nursing care.

The child   For the child the advantage of care by parents is to maintain the comfort and security with his or her parent's presence. McClure and Ryburn as far back as 1969 saw the many advantages for the child not least of all improved child care at home and better health care for the whole family. In 1947, in the UK, Spence clearly took a similar view when he observed that by far the greater part of sick children's nursing is already done in the home and it is therefore logical that it should be continued in hospital. We have been very slow to take this idea on board, but Casey (1988) does accept the concept when she writes about a parent being the expert on his or her own child.

Sainsbury *et al* (1986) claim that it reduces the emotional stress on the child and the family, shortens the period in hospital and because health education is better, may decrease the likelihood of re-admission.

Vass Fore and Holmes (1983) feel that care by parents encourages positive parent/child interaction, and of course as Sainsbury *et al* (1986) argue the child's need for his or her parents is greatest when he or she is ill; and the sicker the child is the more constantly he or she requires his or her parents.

It could also be argued that the more knowledgeable parents are and the more responsibility they take for the child's care the more they feel in control. This must then help to diminish the child's anxiety.

Cleary *et al* (1986) carried out a structured observational study to monitor the effect of care by parents on the child and found that he or she spent far less time awake alone, cried less and slept less than those who were nursed unaccompanied. Most of their contacts and nearly 90% of their interactions were with family members, especially mothers.

The parent Jennings (1986) when discussing care by parents in America and Canada sees it as promoting mental and physical health for the entire family. It follows, then, as Casey (1988) so rightly points out, that if parents are valued for what they do, it increases their self-confidence. If self-confidence is increased and parents are valued for their contribution, then communication between nurses and parents improves. Cleary (1986) suggests that parents can then relate better to the nurses and feel more comfortable with taking on responsibility. For care by parents to work, then, parents must be prepared to accept responsibility, but nurses must ensure that that responsibility is clarified and that their confidence and competence is also reinforced.

Consolvo (1986) in her study 'Relieving parental anxiety in a care by parent unit' found that mothers showed significantly less anxiety in a situation after the care by parent experience.

Miles and Carter (1985) looked at coping strategies used by parents during their child's hospitalization and found that 92% of the parents questioned, used the coping strategy of 'being near my child as much as possible' and 'believing my child is getting the best care possible'.

Sainsbury *et al* (1986) observe that parents sometimes find it irksome to be with their child in the same cubicle continuously. They may resent nurses caring for their child, they may become bored, and for some nurses they may become quite threatening. The logical solution to these problems is for the parents to be the care-givers for their children.

It could therefore be argued that a care by parent scheme helps to clarify the parents' role, allowing them to feel more in control by actively participating in and taking responsibility for their child's care.

The nurse Jennings (1986) feels that, in order to make a care by parent scheme work, nurses must have a well developed paediatric background and a sensitivity to family needs. She also feels that they should practice primary care to provide education and counselling and to assist with problem solving. This can be seen as a very positive step for nurses who are expanding their role to function at their full professional capacity, as long as they have an orientation to the philosophy of care by parents and are willing to spend the necessary time required to involve parents as actual contributing members of the team.

Monahan and Schade (1985) in their study comparing care by parent and traditional nursing units, ask if the quality of nursing care could be compromised by allowing parents to assume total responsibility for patient care and conclude that it is not. It should be seen rather as a challenge both for the nurse and parents.

The future for care by parents

In her study of care by parents, Evans (1990) found that parents were willing and able to participate in the care of their children, but that in some instances nurses needed to change their attitudes. Nurses have always seen themselves as the primary carer even though this is shared with parents in paediatric nursing. Care by parents can only be successful if nurses do not feel threatened by handing the care over to parents and are able to see themselves in an educational and facilitative role.

It is therefore essential that nurses are given appropriate training so that they understand their new role and find care by parents acceptable. They must also develop a cohesive therapeutic and flexible atmosphere on the unit, which allows successful interaction between nurses and parents. In this way there should be less potential for conflict especially if each person's role and responsibility is clearly defined. Too often in nursing new programmes and philosophies are set up without first defining and structuring a clear plan. Care by parents could be a failure never to be repeated if this is not achieved.

It could also be a failure if parents feel exploited and consideration is not given to their needs. It must never be seen as a cost or time saving exercise and parents must always be given the option to hand over to the nurse at any time without feeling guilty.

All care should be negotiated with parents to reach a mutually satisfactory understanding of how the child's care is managed. At this time also individual variations in the needs and abilities of parents should be assessed and taken into account, so that they are able to trust the nurse and do not feel 'taken for granted'.

In the final analysis it is quite clear that the responsibility for the care of the child rests firmly with the nurse. In a care by parent unit that responsibility is greater because he or she is responsible for other people's actions as well as his or her own. Care by parents is an exciting venture but to be successful it must be carefully managed.

References

Bowlby, J. (1953) *Child Care and the Growth of Love.* Penguin, Harmondsworth.
Casey, A. (1988) Partnership in practice. *Nursing Times,* **84** (44) 66–8.
Cleary, J. *et al* (1986) Parental involvement in the lives of children in hospital. *Archives of diseases in childhood,* **61,** 779–87.
Consolvo, C.A. (1984) Relieving parental anxiety in the care by parent unit. *JOGNN,* **13,** 154–7.
Court, S.D.M. (1976) Committee on Child Health Service: Fit for the Future. HMSO, London.
DHSS (1990 Welfare of children in hospital. HMSO, London.
Evans, M. (1987) Learning to lose fear. *Nursing Times,* **83** (1), 55–6.
Evans, M. (1990) An investigation into the feasibility of parental participation in the nursing care of the child. (Unpublished research project).

Evans, R.G. and Robinson, G.C. (1983) An economic study of cost savings on a care by parent ward. *Medical Care*, **21** (8), 768-82.

Fradd, E. (1988) Achieving new roles. *Nursing Times*, **84** (50), 38–40.

Glasper, A. (1990) Emancipation of parents. *Nursing Standard*, **4** (22).

Jennings, K. (1986) Helping them face tomorrow *Nursing Times*, **82**, 33–5.

McLure, M.J. and Ryburn, A.C. (1969) Care by parent unit. *American Journal of Nursing*, **70**, 2148–52.

Miles, M.S. and Carter, M.C. (1985) Coping strategies used by parents during their childs hospitalization in an ICU. *CHC*, Summer, **14** (1), 14–21.

Monahan, G.H. and Schkade, J.K. (1985) Comparing care by parent and traditional nursing units. *Paediatric Nursing*, **11**, 463–8.

Oberlander, R. (1980) Parent care units bring home to the hospital. *Hospitals*, **54**, 81–5.

Platt, H. (1959) Welfare of children in hospital. DHSS, London.

Robertson, J. (1958) Young Children in Hospital. Tavistock, London.

Sainsbury, C.P.Q. *et al* (1986) Care by parents of their children in hospital. *Archives of Disease in Childhood*, **61**, 612–5.

Spence, J.C. (1947) The care of children in hospital. *British Medical Journal*, **1**, 125–30.

Vass Fore, C. and Holmes, S.S. (1983) A care by parent unit re-visited. *MCN*, **8**, 408–10.

Webb, N., Hull D. and Madeley, R. (1985) Care by parents in hospital. *British Medical Journal*, **291**, 176–7.

39

How well do we perform? Parents' perceptions of paediatric care

Margaret Ball, BN, RGN
Teaching Assistant, Department of Nursing Studies

Alan Glasper, BA, RGN, RSCN, ONC, CertEd, RNT
Professor of Nursing Studies

Paul Yerrell, BSc, PhD
Visiting Fellow, Department of Nursing Studies, all at the University of Southampton

Towards the end of 1987, staff on the Paediatric Unit at Southampton General Hospital were worried by staff shortages and associated low morale. There were fears that standards of care could be falling, so there developed a keen interest to measure the quality of care on the unit.

Quality is defined by Roberts (1975) as a grade of goodness, ie it is a measurement. Quality assurance is a process of looking at a given situation and appraising it against a measure or a set standard. In the nursing context this enables nurses to promise and maintain a set standard of care. Setting standards is a vital part in this process which the RCN is pursuing with its standards of care project (Kitson, 1988).

Assessing quality of care

One of the most frequently used frameworks for looking at quality of care is that developed by Donabedian (1976). This is based on three distinct, but interrelated factors; structure, process and outcome. Structure looks at the environmental and resource items and their organisation. Process refers to the planning and delivery of the nursing interventions and outcome is concerned with the result of care. Kitson (1988) has devised a model which can be used to look at these three aspects. She describes the process of quality assurance as cyclic, consisting of describing the problem, measuring it and then taking action. Each of these areas can then be broken down into more specific steps (Figure 1). As the process is cyclic it can be entered at any point.

Quality assurance is a subject very much in vogue. Many tools have been developed, such as Monitor, which has been adapted from an American version by Goldstone (1983). Some of these are being used in the clinical setting to evaluate and measure quality of care. In America, quality assurance programmes are much more developed than ours, partly because of their private health care system, in which insurance companies demand to know standards of care, but also because of their higher levels of medical litigation. In the UK there has been an increasing recognition of the need for work on quality, which has developed for numerous reasons. Of particular influence has been the implementation of Griffiths style management with its emphasis on cost effectiveness. Also, the public are becoming more medically aware, and their expectations of the health services are increasing.

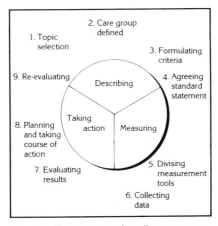

Figure 1. The process of quality assurance.

Quality assurance in paediatrics

Little work has been done on quality assurance in the paediatric field. Some previous work by Maddison (1977) highlighted the importance of seeking the opinion of consumers. Maddison believes parental opinion is most valid in paediatrics in that it reflects that of the child. She further states that she would like to see a grading system for evaluating paediatric wards similar to the stars used to grade hotels. This grade would be strongly influenced by the degree of emotional support offered to children and their parents.

Brykczynska (1987) points out that nurses must work with the child and family, not against them or in spite of them. The child should be viewed as a partner in care, and further work to ascertain children's perceptions of their own care be undertaken.

For the purposes of this pilot study in addressing the staff's worries about care, it was decided to ascertain parental views on the quality of their children's nursing care. This was seen as a way of identifying problems upon which standards of care may be set and further quality work carried out. Although parental opinion is one way of measuring quality of care, it has limitations, because parents' perceptions only relate to perceived quality of care. These do not take into account actual outcome or necessarily reflect the standards of the nursing staff.

The tool chosen to do this was a questionnaire based on some work done at the Hospital for Sick Children in Toronto. It consists of some open-ended questions and some forced choice Likert scale questions in which parents are asked to strongly agree, agree, disagree or strongly disagree to numerous statements (Figure 2). The questionnaire looks at many areas of paediatric nursing care and covers aspects of structure, process and outcome.

For the following statements please check the response which most closely reflects your opinion.	1 Strongly Disagree	2 Disagree	3 Agree	4 Strongly Agree
1. I received consistent information/instructions from each nurse caring for my child during the hospital stay.				
2. I was given adequate information about my child's ward.				
3. I received no information about hospital rules and procedures that might have applied to my family and me.				
4. The nurses always responded to my requests promptly.				
5. The nurses and I discussed how my child's illness or hospitalisation would affect me and my family.				
6. The nurses always asked if I understood what the doctor told me.				
7. I always had trouble getting a nurse when I needed one.				
8. The nurses asked me what I would like to know about my child's illness or hospitalisation.				
9. I feel confident in the nurses caring for my child.				
10. The nurses protected my child's privacy.				
11. I feel confident that I can manage my child's care at home after discharge.				
12. All the nurses caring for my child were familiar with the care he/she needed.				
13. The nurses fully involved me in the planning of my child's nursing care and in the writing of the care plan.				
14. I had to answer a lot of the same questions about my child's needs many times.				
15. If my child was fearful or anxious during any procedures the nurse attempted to reassure, comfort and calm him/her.				
16. I feel the nurses would be willing to stay with my child if he/she was worried or upset about something.				
17. The nurses talked with me and my family about what we could expect to happen during my child's hospitalisation.				
18. I received adequate information about tests and procedures from my child's nurses.				
19. My child received explanation from the nurse that he/she could understand before any procedure was started.				
20. The nurses never asked me how I would prefer my child's care to be carried out.				
21. The nurses helped me feel comfortable in participating in my child's care.				
22. The nurses attended to my child's likes and dislikes as best they could.				
23. The nurses showed genuine interest and concern for my child.				
24. I felt comfortable asking the nurses any questions.				

25. Did you stay with your child during the hospital admission?   YES/NO

   If Yes, was it?:   a) on the ward
                     b) in a cubicle
                     c) in Victoria House?

26. What in your opinion was most helpful to you during the period of time your child was in hospital? Please comment:

27. What could have made the hospital stay better for you as a parent/guardian? Please comment:

28. How would you rate your child's nursing care on this ward.
   A Excellent   C Fair
   B Good   D Poor

29. Date today ....

Your additional comments would be most welcome. Thank you.

Figure 2. The questionnaire (adapted with kind permission of the Hospital for Sick Children, Toronto).

A recent article by Ledwith (1988) notes the recent popularity of consumer surveys in the NHS but emphasises that these should look at the quality of information and support, not just overall patient satisfaction. A single criteria to measure quality may be suited to commercial organisations, but is not sufficient in health care. Work on interpersonal communication has shown communication processes and information levels in the health service have a direct effect on consumer satisfaction. The questionnaire was designed to explore these areas.

The effect of staff-client relationships

Barbarin and Chesler (1984) commented that in areas where staff-client relationships are good, quality of care was better than in those where interpersonal relationships were poor. Their study found respect for medical staff strongly related to parents' perceptions of the transmission of information and their evaluation of the staff's technical competence. Francis et al (1969) found mothers were more likely to comply with treatment when staff were understanding, warm and friendly.

Sheridan (1975) has pointed out that children honour those people who tell the truth about procedures, especially where pain is involved. Good communication helps to minimise the disturbance caused by hospital admission. Other work has found parents of hospitalised children to be highly motivated learners (Aufhauser and Lesh, 1973) who then take information to the community where it is most needed.

The questionnaire was administered to the parents of the first 10 children discharged from each of four paediatric wards in the last week of January 1988. Ward clerks were felt to be the best people to administer them, being the most neutral people on the wards with no direct care input. Complete anonymity was guaranteed and the final sample number was 35; five questionnaires were incompletely answered or not returned.

Results of the survey

Overall the results of the questionnaire demonstrated that parents were satisfied with the care they and their children received. Despite the inherent 'halo' effect commonly seen with this type of research, much valuable data was obtained. Only 8.1 per cent described their child's care as fair, while the remaining 91.4 per cent described it as excellent or good (60 per cent excellent; 31.4 per cent good).

Parents particularly liked being able to stay with their children in hospital and 75.9 per cent of the sample were resident during their child's admission. Written comments revealed that parents greatly appreciated the relaxed atmosphere found on the wards, and many were delighted with the play facilities on offer. All respondents felt they could manage their child's care at home following discharge.

The results did highlight some areas of care where parents were not fully satisfied. Several questions were specifically targeted at information-giving, and the results show there is a need for more information to be given to parents; 33.4 per cent indicated that nursing staff did not ask them if they understood what the doctor had told them and a small number said they did not receive adequate information about the ward or about tests and procedures (11.4 per cent). Some parents (8.6 per cent) felt that information given to them was not always consistent and a minority (5.7 per cent) did not feel comfortable asking nurses questions. Several comments in response to the 'open-ended' questions also reflected this need for more information for parents.

The impact of hospitalisation

The impact of hospitalisation on children and families was addressed in several questions. Responses show this is an area where parents are critical: 38.2 per cent felt there was insufficient discussion by nurses on the effect hospitalisation might have on themselves and their families, and a quarter (25.7 per cent) indicated that nurses did not talk to them about what would happen to their children in hospital.

Parents were highly complimentary about their children's nursing care and attitudes among staff. There were some areas, however, where parental expectations were not met: 40 per cent reported that nurses did not involve them in planning care and a similar number reported that nurses never asked them how they would like their child's care to be carried out. The concept of parental involvement in the care of sick children was also highlighted by several comments indicating that parents would like to do more for their children. Two parents specifically reported that the nursing staff did not make them feel comfortable in participating in their child's care while 14.3 per cent believed that some nurses were not familiar with the care their children needed.

A small number of parents reported that nurses did not respond promptly to requests, but believed this was mitigated by the pressure of work. Several commented on the ward environment; some noted that toys and furniture were not very clean. Comments were also received on excessive noise, such as squeaky doors, and such irritations were thought to be controllable. Some parents were concerned about lighting levels. Some said the lights were too bright at night and suggested darker curtains between cubicles, while others felt greater segregation of children into age groups would allow lights to be turned off earlier for younger children.

A few parents wanted to eat with their children and were reluctant to go to the canteen, calling for more eating facilities on the ward. It is interesting that some parents said they wanted tea and coffee facilities when these facilities did exist on all wards.

In conclusion, the majority of parents identified care to be of a good or excellent standard. In respect to information, hospitalisation, parental involvement, and facilities for parents, a minority of parents saw room for improvements. Here we are reminded of Ledwith's reservation that although overall satisfaction is a useful measure, it is not sufficient in the health service.

Addressing parents' concerns

In the interests of the children we care for, we may need to address the concerns highlighted in this work within the financial and manpower constraints imposed upon clinical areas. With regard to information giving, the results encourage nurses to give parents more information both formally and informally. New areas being explored are preadmission programme, a care by parent scheme, ward booklets and discharge information packs. Nurses are also encouraged to examine how to involve parents more fully in their child's care. The advantages of care by parent schemes such as that initiated in Cardiff (Sainsbury et al, 1986) may result in their continued growth and development in the UK.

While responses to the questionnaire indicate areas where nurses could improve care, the task still remains to describe the structure, process and outcome criteria which will allow specific standards to be set, against which a measurement of quality can be made. Restraints of time may well be hindering nurses in this task and perhaps the results of this pilot study will raise awareness and prompt nurses to look at the issues involved.

We should remind ourselves that if we are to promote nursing as a research-based profession, we should be using the plethora of nursing research to help us achieve our goals of identifying problems, setting standards and measuring quality of care. It will be, of course, for each paediatric unit, as they embark on setting standards in relation to the quality of care, to decide what proportion of time they devote to setting and measuring standards in relation to problems evolving from parents' perceptions. Only when practitioners identify a personal commitment to changing practice and recognise the role parents' views might have in identifying where changes are required, will paediatric units become fully self-evaluating.

References

Aufhauser, T.R. and Lesh, D. (1973) Parents need TLC too. *Hospital*, **47**, 8, 88.
Barbarin, O. and Chesler, M.A. (1984) Relationships with the medical staff and aspects of satisfaction with care expressed by parents of chldren with cancer. *Journal of Community Health*, **9**, 4, 302–13.
Brykczynska, G.M. (1987) Ethical issues in paediatric nursing. *Nursing*, **3**, 862–864.
Donabedian, A. (1976) Measures of quality of care. *American Journal of Nursing*, **76**, 2, 186.
Francis, V. *et al* (1969) Gaps in doctor–patient communication response to medical advice. *New England Journal of Medicine*, **280**, 535–540.
Goldstone, L.A. *et al* (1983) Monitor. Newcastle upon Tyne Polytechnic Products Limited.
Kitson, A.L. (1988) Nursing Quality Assurance, Dynamic Standard Setting System. RCN Standards of Care Project, unpublished.
Ledwith, F. (1988) Doing less to achieve more. *Health Service Journal*, **98**, 3088.
Maddison, M. (1977) Consumer survey of paediatric wards. *Australian Nurses' Journal*, **6**, 1, 27–28.

Roberts, I. (1975) Discharged from hospital. Royal College of Nursing, London.
Sainsbury, C.P.Q. *et al* (1986) Care by parents of their children in hospital. *Archives of Disease in Childhood*, **61**, 612–615.
Sheridan, M.S. (1975) Children's feelings about the hospital. *Social Work in Health Care*, **1**, 65–70.

Index

INDEX